Sound Sense

Sound Sense
Living and Learning with Hearing Loss

Sara Laufer Batinovich

Gallaudet University Press
Washington, DC

Gallaudet University Press
Washington, DC 20002
http://gupress.gallaudet.edu

Library of Congress Cataloging-in-Publication Data

Batinovich, Sara Laufer.
  Sound sense : living and learning with hearing loss / Sara Laufer
Batinovich.
     p. cm.
  Includes bibliographical references and index.
  ISBN-13: 978-1-56368-471-5 (pbk. : alk. paper)
  ISBN-10: 1-56368-471-3 (pbk. : alk. paper)
  1. Deafness.   2. Hearing disorders.   3. Hearing aid.   I. Title.

RF290.B38 2010
617.8—dc22   2010035524

For John

What Mr. Watson heard:

"Mr. Watson—
come here—I want
to see you."

Alexander Graham Bell
March 10, 1876

*What a person with a hearing loss
would have heard:*

"Mr. Wa   on—
co e he e—I
wa to ee ou."

Contents

List of Figures

Preface

SOUND SENSE IS a book for people who choose to identify as culturally hearing—people whose primary form of communication is speech and who do not use sign language. This distinction is central to the purpose of this book. Many culturally Deaf individuals prefer not to conform to the mainstream, hearing culture, and they are often steadfast in their preference to use signing—their organic and native language—exclusively as their communication system. The author respects these choices.

This book, in contrast, is predicated on the value of hearing for everyday activities, such as work, education, romantic relationships, and overall health. As such, it is targeted toward people who have lost enough of their hearing to have experienced interference with their daily activities and relationships, and the stresses and hassles that accompany managing these challenges. Whether a person with a hearing loss calls herself or himself "hard of hearing," "hearing impaired," a "person with a hearing loss," or "clinically deaf"—all terms used interchangeably in this book—she or he has chosen to identify with the hearing culture and, as such, has a different set of communication inclinations than someone who chooses to be culturally Deaf.

If you have a hearing loss and are in the working-age population, you have a tough job. Every one of your decisions regarding your occupation, your health, your activities, and your relationships is influenced by your hearing loss. It is not an easy way of life. To be integrated in society, to be fully invested in the hearing world, and to maximize your potential takes a lot of energy, planning, flexibility, and creativity. *Sound Sense* will enable you to help yourself by showing you ways to live a life full of learning, loving, and laughing with a hearing loss. You'll be better able to orchestrate your life's symphony and become the maestro of your goals and dreams.

Acknowledgments

It is not so much cliché as axiomatic to say that I am grateful to the many remarkable souls who have helped me with my research and in my life. I am honored to acknowledge their contributions to this project, and, more importantly, to my life.

Several people generously gave their time, sage opinions, and expertise by providing insightful comments on various sections of this book. Thank you to Janice Chang, Mark P. Ewens, Sherri Fisher, Brad Garrett, David Laufer, Maria Mander, Gabriel Martinez, Tom Piazza, Ruth Sheff, Susan Stoddard, Vivian Walker, Clinton Wong, and Fan-Gang Zeng.

I thank Barbara Kelley for her encouragement, and for her unrelenting commitment to people with hearing loss.

The late Alexander Hivoltze-Jimenez urged me many years ago to write this book. His spirit continues to inspire me to help other people with hearing loss.

It is with admiration that I thank Burton Craige and Alyssa Gsell for being champions of justice.

For his gifted photography and his generous spirit, I thank Joe Buissink.

Crackerjack data and research experts graciously responded to my questions (and more questions) as I researched this material. Thank you to Aurora D'Amico at the U.S. Department of Education/National Center for Education Statistics, David Maack and the government publications staff at the University of Washington Libraries in Seattle and Tacoma, Eric A. Mann and Shu-Chen Peng at the U.S. Food and Drug Administration, and Jada Pelger and Lori Ricigliano at the University of Puget Sound Collins Memorial Library.

I also have been blessed by people who have guided me throughout my career with their professional wisdom and voices of experience. Thank you to Ellen Atlas, Michael Burke, Anthony J. Cascardi, Erik Doxtader, Richard Dulin, Leon Faure, Pete Groeneveld, Gene Hammel, Jennifer Johnson-Hanks, Bob Hasson, John A. Hodges, Mike Hout, Jane Iwamura, Robert K. Jackler, Randy Jordan, Theodore Keeler, Rob Komas, Ron Lee, Michael Mascuch, Carl Mason, Jane Mauldon, Daniel F. Melia, David Nasatir, Laura Lee Norris, Pat Paoli, Roberta Reynolds, Bill Satariano, Linda Scholer, Judith Lawson Selsor, David Stern, Mathew J. Temmerman, Patricia Tollefson, Mary Vencill, Ken Wachter, Nancy Weston, and John Wilmoth.

Many wonderful people have been my cheerleaders over the years. Thank you to Susan Bratton, Chuck Bremberg, Jennifer Bryce, Carl Buising, Kavita Choudhry, Sara Clair, Les and Olga Culver, Anne Danenberg, Brent Fischer, Patricia Frieze, Karen Laufer Gold, Pepper Gregory, Martin Harband, Susan Heartlight, Stu Jones, Leonard Kanner, Kimberly Krantz, Sandy Kurozawa, Trana and Ronnie Labowe, Jan Larky, Nancy Laufer, Ted Laufer, Christophe Lobry-Boulanger, Kai Mander, Porter Merriman, Betty Morey, Kim Nicols, Liz Ozselcuk, Cathy Parks, James Raimondo, Alison J. Rigby, Ronda Rose, Andrea Schall, Dennis Sinor, Paul Soals, Toni and Walter Sosnosky, Sarah Tom, Royden Tonomura, Donnamaie White, Toni Will, Bob and Mary Woolsey, Dave Wong, and Yar.

My editor, Ivey Wallace, is a gift to people with hearing loss and to the publishing world. Thanks, Ivey. I am also grateful to Gallaudet University Press's production and marketing teams: managing editor Deirdre Mullervy; copy editor Michelle Harris; production coordinator Donna Thomas; marketing director Daniel Wallace; and marketing assistant Valencia Simmons.

And finally, I thank my mother, Joyce K. Laufer, and my late father, Charles A. Laufer, for their love and for encouraging me to write from the time that I was old enough to hold a crayon.

Introduction: A Silent Avalanche

THROUGHOUT THE MILLENNIA of human civilization, hearing has been inextricably linked to cultural development and interpersonal engagement. Rituals and ceremonies move forward with dialogues and music. The judicial system relies on spoken testimony in Congressional hearings, criminal trials, and small claims cases. And the evolution of entertainment has been increasingly reliant on sound; from ancient Greek plays to radio, talking films, record albums, television, compact discs, and now MP3 players and audio-based files on the Internet, all of these media depend heavily—or exclusively—on one's sense of hearing.

We spend up to half of each day listening, an activity that engages both sensory perception and cognition.[1] Hearing is a sense that informs us constantly; about one month before birth, fetuses can recognize different voices from the womb.[2] Sound also enriches everyday experiences by creating multisensory pleasure, such as the crunching of soft snow when we pack it into balls, or the crashing of waves that spray salty mist on us at the beach on a hot summer's day.

The abilities to speak and to hear have long been regarded as vital to living a full existence. In the past, the U.S. Census Bureau categorized people who did not have these abilities along with people who had intellectual disabilities,[3] and definitions of "deaf" in *The Oxford English Dictionary* include the terms inattentive, dull, stupid, absurd, numb, hollow, unproductive, and barren.[4] Alexander Graham Bell (yes, the inventor of the telephone) promoted eugenic practices and discouraged people who were Deaf from intermarrying and having children in order to create a better society with fewer "undesirables."[5]

1

Throughout history, the need to hear has been regarded as an essential part of being human. Words such as audience, audiology, audible, audition, and auditor are all derived from the Latin *audire*, meaning "to hear." For example, the first definition of "audience" in *The Oxford English Dictionary* is "the action of hearing; attention to what is spoken."[6] All through our lives, we participate as members of an audience more than we sleep or work.[7]

When a person loses all or some ability to hear, she or he loses far more than conversational skills. Work, relationships, leisure activities, health care, and self-perception are all influenced, and every decision a person with a hearing loss makes for the rest of her or his life will be affected by this chronic condition. A hard of hearing person cannot assume anything, least of all the impact that the change from hearing well to hearing poorly has on one's life.

This change is slow and subtle for most people. More than four out of five (82 percent) people between the ages of 18 and 66 notice a gradual decline in their hearing, not a sudden drop. Also, relatively few people are born hard of hearing or develop this disability in their retirement years; among working-age adults with permanent hearing loss, 77 percent experienced the onset of their losses after they were teenagers.[8] The prevalence of hearing loss is highest among older adults. But the 46-year-olds of today are the 66-year-olds of 2030, and undiagnosed or untreated hearing loss in young adult or middle age will likely have a negative effect for decades.

A Demographer with Hearing Loss

If comfort can be found in numbers, people with hearing loss have plenty of company. Nearly one out of every eight people between the ages of 18 and 66 in the United States has a hearing loss. These more than twenty-three million adults—12 percent of the working-age population—comprise a group nearly as big as the population of Texas. And it is likely that this number is low, because 27 percent of working-age men and 31 percent of working-age women have never had a hearing test.[9] Hearing loss affects more non-elderly adults than diabetes, coronary heart disease, or ulcers.[10] By the year 2050, if the proportion of the population with hearing loss remains constant, more than 29 million Americans in the working-age group will be hard of hearing.[11]

I am already one of them. Since I first noticed a problem with my hearing when I was 13 years old—my sister did not understand why I could not hear the "dinger" on the oven when I baked chocolate chip cookies—I have been grappling with the same issues as my hearing impaired brethren. From getting and paying for hearing aids to planning my wedding so that I could hear with my new cochlear implant, and from educating other people in line at the post office about my hearing service dog to deciding what to disclose about my hearing loss in job interviews, I face many of the same challenges as millions of others. I try to regard these situations as opportunities for growth; I don't always succeed, but I usually enjoy the process.

Along the way, I became a demographer specializing in hearing health care policy research. This trajectory was unexpected; not once during my childhood did I say to my parents, "When I grow up, I want to be a demographer!" In fact, I started out as a musician, starting with piano lessons at age seven, and then I played woodwinds all through junior and senior high school. I miss that part of my life, but I still cherish the gifts that music gave me even now that I am clinically deaf. However weird it sounds, I remain an auditory learner and have a memory based on sounds that has let me adapt to life's changes with some extra layers of sensory prosperity.

While in school and at work, when dating online, and while striving to develop and maintain healthy friendships and relationships, the center of my life has moved to a very different place from where it was when my hearing was normal. This additional perspective has made me more whole rather than less complete, and more sensitive to others rather than less understanding.

I realized many years ago that many of the barriers that sometimes keep me from achieving my goals are those that I erect myself, or have not yet removed. It takes a lot of work to manage a hearing loss in the hearing world. It can be simultaneously exhausting and exhilarating to navigate and negotiate in a noisy world, but it sure is worth the effort. When I got on my own side, a lot of magic happened without any need for a wand or a fairy godmother.

The importance of being your own best advocate cannot be underestimated. It takes persistence and a strong sense of self. It also means using available resources to stand up to discrimination when necessary. For instance, when I went back to college as a nontraditional re-entry student newly fitted with hearing aids, I had to grapple with campus administrators who were digging in their heels to avoid complying with the then-new Americans with Disabilities Act. It was a harsh lesson in how to get people to do the right (and legal) thing, when they wanted nothing more than for me to just go away.

During that time, I read Alice Walker's *Possessing the Secret of Joy*. While the circumstances in the novel were different, its message "RESISTANCE IS THE SECRET OF JOY!"[12] resonated within me, and I have remembered those words when faced with ignorance or flat-out discrimination that threatened to prevent me from working, going to school, or taking my hearing dog into a store. In the pages that follow, some of my best and worst moments since losing my hearing will, I hope, inform parts of your own life, and give you tips, tools, and techniques for not just surviving, but thriving.

I wish I had known the information in this book when my hearing loss started to accelerate in my late teens. It was a scary and sobering time. I knew nothing about getting hearing aids, and I had never heard of assistive devices. When I was able to afford my first pair of hearing aids at age 28, the sticker shock, the discombobulated purchase process, and the repeated visits to my doctor's and audiologist's offices were frustrating in their inefficiency. It was both vindicating and depressing to read in a recent issue of *Consumer Reports* that my dissatisfaction with the hearing health care delivery system is not uncommon. Gaps in product information, fitting errors, and the cost of hearing aids were frequent predicaments documented by *Consumer Reports*.[13] These systemic problems need to be considered as possible causes of low hearing aid use among the hard of hearing population: Among adults of all ages (including older adults), about one in six—not quite 17 percent—people with hearing loss wears hearing aids.[14]

Hearing Loss in the Working Ages

Even fewer adults under age 67 wear hearing aids: About one in fourteen—7 percent—working-age adults with hearing loss uses these devices.[15] In this age group, only 6 percent of men and 9 percent of women with a hearing loss have had a hearing aid recommended by a health care professional.[16] Cochlear implants, which are surgically implanted hearing prosthetics used by people who have severe and profound hearing loss, are not often used by people in the working ages; about 50 working-age adults with a profound hearing loss per 10,000 got a cochlear implant in 2001,[17] and some 41,500 adults had been implanted in the United States as of April 2009.[18] The devices were first approved for use in the United States in 1984.[19]

A considerable unmet need exists for information about hearing loss, hearing health care, life management strategies, and overall health for people in the working-age group. If provided, this information may increase the access to and use of hearing health care. Many books describe ways to manage hearing loss in children and older adults and offer expert guidance on choosing a hearing aid. But few resources exist to help those in the longest phase of the life cycle—the income earning years—with the everyday challenges, attributes, and unique needs of this diverse and dynamic population.

Hearing health care tends to be focused on patients who are young and old, but not in their working years. It is common, for example, to see toys and games in an audiologist's testing booth and hearing aid brochures featuring photographs of mature adults in the waiting room. People with hearing loss also have different technology and communications needs from the needs of people with visual impairments, mobility impairments, or other disabilities.

I find two key reasons why hearing loss is eclipsed as a condition warranting more attention in the working-age group. First, it is not a "marquee" condition that grabs headlines, such as the H1N1 virus. While it shares its chronic nature with other conditions, and its stigma with obesity and HIV, on its own a hearing impairment is seldom fatal or a covered benefit of mainstream health insurance (an explanation for this frequent benefit exclusion is in chapter 6), as are most other chronic conditions. The effects of the stigma associated with hearing impairment are powerful—the disability is easy to deny, and comfortable to ignore. Interestingly, hearing loss is often associated with several other serious health conditions, including diabetes; recent research suggests that "diabetes might affect the vasculature and neural system of the inner ear, leading to hearing impairment."[20] Analyses presented in chapter 5 show higher prevalence rates of diabetes in nonelderly adults with hearing loss relative to nonelderly adults with excellent or good hearing, along with the associations of hearing loss with depression, asthma, hypertension, and—a big surprise—falls.

Second, hearing loss can be an expensive condition that requires a long-term investment of time and money. Unlike correcting vision by having laser surgery or by getting a new pair of glasses, and unlike fixing a cavity by getting a filling, managing hearing loss takes substantial effort in learning how to hear and to communicate better after paying a lot of money for hearing aids. Everyone with a hearing loss needs the cooperation and compassion of friends, relatives, and coworkers to be successful in her or his health improvement efforts, so the effort extends beyond the individual. At times, those obligations can be exasperating and cumbersome.

However, the benefits of hearing health care—specifically, hearing aids—are well documented in the literature, although most research focuses on the benefits among the elderly. One study found that four out of five participants experienced a "significant benefit from the hearing aid use."[21] Another project found that hearing aids improved psychosocial issues including anxiety and depression, and self-reliance resulting from hearing loss in adults.[22] While a task force within the American Academy of Audiology—an organization of audiologists with an obvious interest in increasing hearing aid sales—conducted that study, the results are consistent with the original analysis on depression and hearing aids in chapter 5 that shows that working-age people who wear hearing aids have lower rates of depression than working-age people with hearing loss who do not wear hearing aids.

Almost 97 percent of the hearing aids sold in the United States use sophisticated digital technology,[23] and regardless of type the average price of one hearing aid is $1,676, with a range of $900 to $3,400 per aid.[24] Digital aids are more expensive than aids using older analog technology, but research indicates that the pricier devices may not be necessary for many people from a medical standpoint, although personal preference may drive the higher satisfaction rates found for the digital products.[25] In other words, take that first step and get a well-fitted hearing aid, which can provide substantial benefit[26] without costing thousands of dollars.

However, the most often cited reason for not purchasing a hearing aid is cost: Among the nonelderly adult population with hearing loss, 32 percent of men and 49 percent of women report that they do not use a hearing aid because the devices are too expensive.[27] This barrier to care is critical to address, given the associations between hearing loss and the comorbid conditions in working-age adults noted earlier.

Other countries, including Germany, Switzerland, and the United Kingdom, have acknowledged the importance of hearing health care for their working-age populations by providing partial or full benefits to nonelderly adults for hearing aids, with some restrictions on the types of devices covered. Public insurance in Germany pays a fixed amount for hearing aids, and dispensers must provide service for the aids for five years. Patients can buy more expensive products and pay the difference out-of-pocket. In Switzerland, privately funded mandatory insurance pays the full cost of hearing aids and care after purchase; the type of aid provided is determined by the listening requirements of the patient. As in Germany, the person with a hearing loss can purchase costlier amplification and pay the amount above the reimbursement limit. The National Health Service (NHS) in the United Kingdom provides hearing aids free of charge, although there are waiting lists.[28] The NHS has reduced waiting times recently, with 99 percent of hearing-health consumers receiving care within eighteen weeks.[29]

New Findings

The analyses that follow highlight the working-age group population of adults under age 67. While traditionally the nonelderly age category has been considered to be ages 18–64, most people now working will not reach retirement until their 67th birthdays. (For people born in or after 1960, full Social Security benefits will not be available until age 67.) Given the recent economic downturn and the likelihood that more people will be working longer, research findings using ages 18–66 provide a more accurate picture of this segment.

The National Health Interview Survey (NHIS) provides the data for most of the charts and graphs. A household health survey, the NHIS has been administered annually in the United States since 1957. While questions and sample sizes have changed over the years, the fundamental purpose of the NHIS is to take an annual snapshot of the health of Americans of all ages, using self-reported information. The U.S. Census Bureau collects the data through in-person interviews in the respondents' homes and provides data files of the survey responses that are available for analysis on the National Center for Health Statistics Web site.

The three hearing loss categories in this book correspond to the NHIS response choices for hearing ability *without hearing aids or equipment used for hearing*. The first category is comprised of people who self-reported "excellent" or "good" hearing, the second category includes those who self-reported "a little trouble hearing," and the third category is made up of respondents who self-reported "moderate trouble" or "a lot of trouble" hearing. A few findings use two hearing categories instead of three—first, those with excellent or good hearing, and second, those with any trouble hearing. Two categories instead of three are used when the number of respondents for a particular question is too low to stratify into three groups. Appendix A has more details about the NHIS, including a link to the survey Web site.

If you are allergic to math, fear not! You do not need training in statistics to read and use the charts and tables in this book. Let's get started.

The Demography of Hearing Loss

Figure 1 shows a breakdown by age of working-age people with hearing loss. Out of everyone ages 18–66 with any trouble hearing, more than half (55 percent) are 50–66 years old, slightly more than one third (36 percent) are 30–49 years old, and 9 percent are 18–29 years old. Since hearing loss increases with age, these findings are not surprising, but it is worth noting that, in absolute terms, the 45 percent of people with hearing loss younger than 50 years old make up a group of more than ten million people, as large as the population of Michigan.

While health care professionals do not often recommend the use of hearing health care to nonelderly adults, as shown above,

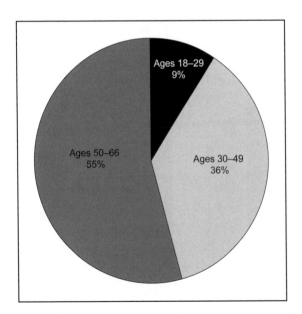

Figure 1. Hearing loss by age category in the working-age population, United States, 2008. *Refused to answer, not ascertained, and don't know responses were excluded.*

once people ages 18–66 get hearing aids, they tend to use them often. Just under 50 responded that they have always used their hearing aid in the past year, while 37 percent answered that they have usually used their devices, or have used them about half the time, in the past year.[30]

The twenty-three million working-age people with hearing loss show variations in several other demographic and social groups. The following figures show hearing loss disparities by age group and sex, marital status, race and ethnicity, native and foreign-born status, and employment.

Figure 2 shows that among working-age adults who have excellent or good hearing, a higher proportion are women (52 percent)

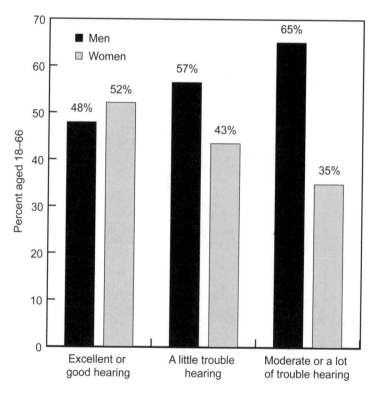

Figure 2. Hearing status by sex, ages 18–66, United States, 2008. *Refused to answer, not ascertained, and don't know responses were excluded.*

than men (48 percent). The gender balance shifts among those with trouble hearing, however. People ages 18–66 with a little trouble hearing are more likely to be men (57 percent) than women (43 percent), and the difference becomes more pronounced in people with moderate or a lot of trouble hearing, among whom almost two out of three (65 percent) are men, and about one in three (35 percent) are women. The differences may be partially explained by the higher noise exposure that men experience compared to women. Men may also be more likely to report a hearing loss.

Marital Status

As figure 3 shows, among working-age adults with excellent or good hearing, 63 percent are married or living with a partner, 11 percent are divorced or separated, and 26 percent have never been married. In contrast, 73 percent of people with any trouble hearing are married or living with a partner, 16 percent are divorced or separated, and 11 percent have never been married. It is interesting to note that people ages 18–66 with hearing loss are more likely to be in partnerships, and are more likely to have their partnerships end before death, than are their better-hearing counterparts. The higher rate of marriage and lower rate of "never-marrieds" among people with hearing loss may be due in part to age, since more older people have hearing loss, or perhaps some people with hearing loss are more likely to seek out unions for stability and assistance than do people with better hearing. Reasons for these differences, and for the higher dissolution rates among people with hearing loss, would be interesting to explore further.

Race/Ethnicity

Figure 4 illustrates differences in hearing loss by race and ethnicity. In the working-age group sorted by race, people of Asian descent report having a hearing loss less frequently than any other racial group (4 percent), and people identifying as being multiple race have the highest rates of hearing loss (15 percent). Six percent of Hispanics, 6 percent of Blacks, and 13 percent of Whites are hard of hearing.

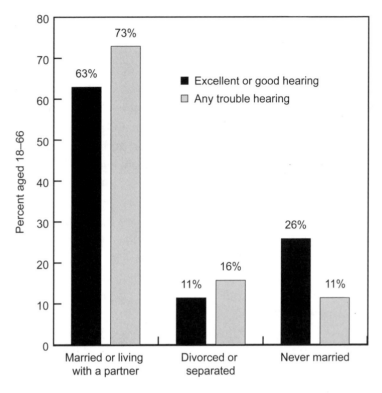

Figure 3. Marital status by hearing category, ages 18-66, United States, 2008. *Respondents were ages 18–66, excluding widows and widowers who comprised a very small percentage of the working-age group in this survey. The "married" category included spouses living in the same or different households, and respondents living with partners. Refused to answer, not ascertained, don't know, and unknown responses were excluded.*

Possible barriers to hearing health care among older Black adults include a dearth of culturally appropriate information about the subject, a lack of interest in getting hearing aids, and insufficient awareness about hearing resources among their primary care physicians.[31] It is plausible that cultural practices and attitudes are partially responsible for the perceived differences in hearing loss prevalence among younger adults and other races or

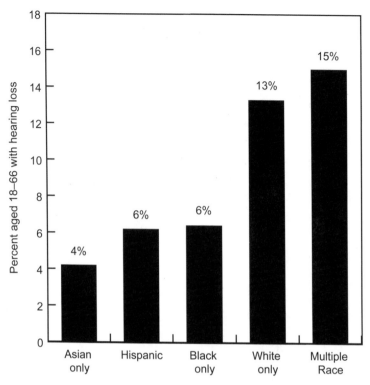

Figure 4. Hearing loss by race and ethnicity, ages 18–66, United States, 2008. *Categories determined by the Office of Management and Budget (OMB). The American Indian/Alaska Native and "not releasable" categories are not shown because of too few responses to be statistically valid. Refused to answer, not ascertained, and don't know responses were excluded. Asian, Black, White, and Multiple Race categories are "races" according to OMB, and the Hispanic category is an "ethnicity."*

ethnicities. Members of some groups may be less likely to disclose or acknowledge a hearing loss.

Do the disparities in hearing loss represent true differences in the prevalence of the condition, or do they illustrate different mores and values? The answers will help ensure that potentially underserved population segments receive better outreach and care. Educational resources about noise-induced hearing loss targeted to people in different racial or ethnic groups—and distinct age groups—have been found to be more effective than generic information.[32]

Native and Foreign-born

More than twice as many working-age people born in the United States report having a hearing loss compared to the foreign-born living in the United States (13 percent versus 5 percent), as shown in figure 5. As with race and ethnicity differences, some cultural factors may be driving the disparities. Biological differences are unlikely to be responsible for the disparities, so looking at the reasons that make people more or less likely to acknowledge a

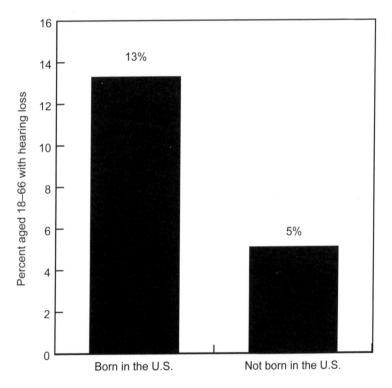

Figure 5. Hearing loss by native or foreign-born status, ages 18–66, United States, 2008. *Refused to answer, not ascertained, and don't know responses were excluded.*

hearing loss may lead to better ways to provide health care services to minority and foreign-born populations.

Employment

Women have lower employment rates than men regardless of hearing ability. Figure 6 shows that, out of all people ages 18–49 with excellent or good hearing, 82 percent of men and 71 percent of women are working. Among younger working-age adults with a little trouble hearing, 84 percent of men and 71 percent of women are working. Both men and women with moderate or a

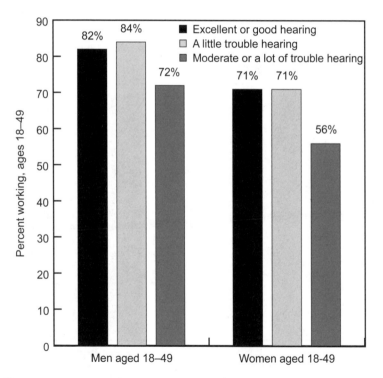

Figure 6. Percentage of people working, by hearing ability and sex, ages 18-49, United States, 2008. *Working is defined as working for pay the week before the survey or having a job but not at work during that week (for example, on vacation or taking sick time). Refused to answer, not ascertained, and don't know responses excluded.*

lot of trouble hearing have appreciably lower employment rates than their counterparts with better hearing throughout the working ages, with the exception of women ages 50–66 (see figure 7); just over half of women in this age group with any hearing loss are working (52 percent with the greatest difficulty hearing, and a negligibly different 51 percent with a little trouble hearing).

Nearly half of all women with moderate or a lot of trouble hearing, regardless of age, and almost half of men ages 50–66 with moderate or a lot of trouble hearing, are not working. Being

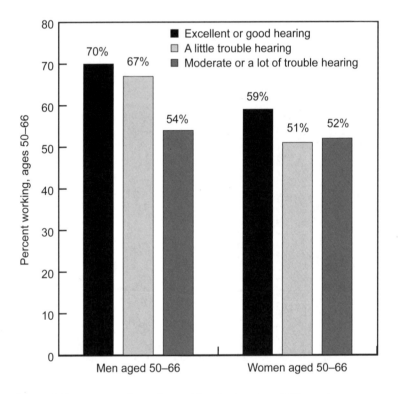

Figure 7. Percentage of people working, by hearing ability and sex, ages 50-66, United States, 2008. *Working is defined as working for pay the week before the survey or having a job but not at work during that week (for example, on vacation or taking sick time). Refused to answer, not ascertained, and don't know responses excluded.*

disabled was cited as the main reason for not working by 21 percent of people with excellent or good hearing, by 37 percent of people with a little trouble hearing, and by 45 percent of people with moderate or a lot of trouble hearing (other main reasons for not working included taking care of the house or family, going to school, and being retired).[33]

The individual and societal benefits of work include opportunities for immediate income, higher social status, a greater sense of personal worth, and stronger connections to family and friends.[34] These benefits are important effects of a successfully managed hearing loss. In addition, people who are economically self-sufficient have the potential to save money for retirement and to reduce or eliminate dependence on entitlement programs. Since Social Security retirement benefits are calculated for each individual based upon that person's earnings history,[35] higher earned income over the worker's lifetime can result in a higher monthly Social Security benefit during the golden years.

Causes of Hearing Loss

As shown in figures 8 and 9, 45 percent of hearing loss in men and 17 percent of hearing loss in women stems from everyday noise exposure. Much of that damage can be prevented through avoiding the noise or by using ear protection. Women attribute hearing loss to the aging process twice as much men (24 percent of women versus 12 percent of men), and many more men than women (13 percent versus 3 percent) attribute their hearing impairment to loud, sudden noises such as gunfire.

Noise in the Working Ages

The dangers of too much noise go beyond causing hearing loss; excess noise has been implicated in conditions ranging from heart disease and hypertension to sleep deprivation and consequent problems with immune system functioning.[36]

Among people ages 18–66 who have ever worked, 25 percent—some 45 million adults—have been exposed to loud noise at work for at least four hours a day, several days a week. Half of

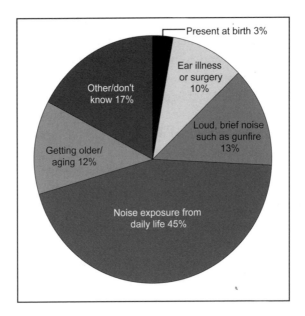

Present at birth 3%
Ear illness or surgery 10%
Other/don't know 17%
Loud, brief noise such as gunfire 13%
Getting older/ aging 12%
Noise exposure from daily life 45%

Figure 8. Causes of hearing loss among working-age men, United States, 2007. *Noise exposure from daily life includes appliances, machinery, loud music, and related everyday sounds. Refused to answer, not ascertained, and don't know responses excluded.*

this group experienced substantial noise exposure on the job in the twelve months prior to the survey, and more than one in three—36 percent—with this recent noise exposure never wore ear protection such as ear plugs or muffs at work during the same period. Among everyone in the working ages who has experienced a minimum of four hours of noise on the job for several days a week, more than four out of ten—41 percent—have been exposed to this level of on-the-job noise for at least ten years.[37]

Leisure-time noise exposure also is pervasive during the working ages. Almost one in four working-age adults—47 million people ages 18–66, or 24 percent—has been exposed to loud noises away from work at least once a month for one year in his or her life, including noise from household appliances, loud music, and power tools. Among everyone in this group, 83 percent have been

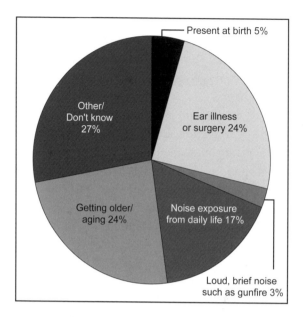

Figure 9. Causes of hearing loss among working-age women, United States, 2007. *Noise exposure from daily life includes appliances, machinery, loud music, and related everyday sounds. Refused to answer, not ascertained, and don't know responses excluded.*

exposed to leisure-time noise in the past twelve months, and more than six out of ten (64 percent) never wore ear protection during this recent noise exposure.[38]

Hearing loss among military personnel is also a huge concern. Noise from bombs, explosives, and gunfire has made more than 58,000 troops who have served in Afghanistan and Iraq eligible for disability benefits resulting from their hearing losses, and almost 70,000 have combat-related tinnitus (a ringing or roaring in the ears). CBS News reports that this extreme noise exposure has made "hearing damage . . . the No. 1 disability in the fight against terror, according to the Department of Veterans Affairs," with blasts in battles reaching 183 decibels.[39] Among the working-age population with Veterans Affairs (VA) health coverage, 32 percent have trouble hearing. In contrast, among the entire working-age population in the United States, 12 percent have trouble hearing.[40] The VA pro-vides veterans as young as 18 with hearing aids; more information about hearing health care for veterans can be found in chapter 3.

Tinnitus

Tinnitus is far more common in people with hearing loss than it is in people with better hearing. A difficult condition to manage, few treatment options are available for tinnitus sufferers and success with those methods varies. No cure is imminent. Figure 10 shows the disparities in tinnitus prevalence by sex and hearing ability.

Just under 6 percent of both men and women with excellent or good hearing report having had tinnitus symptoms lasting at

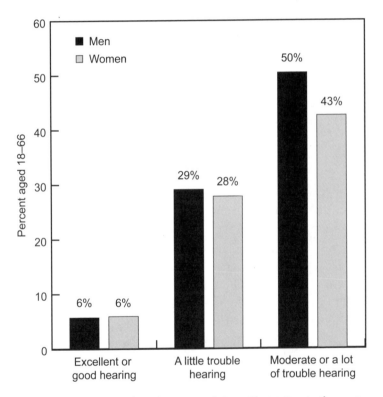

Figure 10. Percentage of working-age adults with tinnitus in the past 12 months, by sex and hearing ability, United States, 2008. *Refused to answer, not ascertained, and don't know responses excluded.*

least five minutes one or more times in the twelve months prior to the survey. Only a little trouble hearing, though, is associated with tinnitus rates almost five times higher (29 percent of men and 28 percent of women), while half of working-age men and more than four in ten women (43 percent) with moderate or a lot of trouble hearing have tinnitus.

Some people ages 18–66 have tinnitus solely after exposure to loud music or sounds, and others experience it when trying to go to sleep, as shown in table 1.[41] About one in six people with better hearing (18 percent) has tinnitus *only* after exposure to loud sounds, 14 percent of people with a little trouble hearing experience ringing in this situation, and 9 percent of people with moderate or a lot of trouble hearing have tinnitus accompanying noise exposure. More than one third of people with excellent or good hearing (35 percent) hear ringing when going to sleep, while more than four in ten people with a little trouble hearing (43 percent) and almost half (48 percent) of people with the most trouble hearing have these symptoms at bedtime. Loud stimuli trigger tinnitus in people with excellent or good hearing more than in people with any hearing trouble, but people with better hearing are less affected by the ringing in their ears when going to sleep.

Table 1. Percentage of people ages 18-66 experiencing tinnitus after loud music or when going to sleep, by hearing ability, United States, 2008. *Respondents experiencing tinnitus after loud music do not report having tinnitus at other times. All respondents to the questions about loud music and sleep had experienced tinnitus symptoms in the 12 months before the survey.*

	Excellent or good hearing	A little trouble hearing	Moderate or a lot of trouble hearing
Only after loud music or sounds	18%	14%	9%
When going to sleep	35%	43%	48%

Source: Author calculations of 2008 National Health Interview Survey data.

Note: Refused and don't know responses excluded.

Promising research in tinnitus includes a project to transmit low-frequency sounds into an MP3 player worn by a person with tinnitus, to mitigate the ringing. The investigator, Dr. Fan-Gang Zeng at the University of California, Irvine, has had encouraging success rates in experimental testing, with roughly 80 percent of study participants experiencing relief from their symptoms.[42]

Hearing Loss Research

Researchers are making progress to cure hearing loss, albeit slowly and with varying degrees of success. Irreparable damage to the delicate hair cells or auditory nerve cells that enable hearing causes over 90 percent of hearing impairment. Scientists at the National Institutes of Health are expanding their theories of hair-cell regeneration based on earlier encouraging findings, with the goal of catalyzing the regeneration of these essential components of the auditory system. The prevention of hearing loss by better understanding the biological system driving the destruction of auditory functioning is also an important area of study.[43] The Institute of Medicine and the World Health Organization have also identified hearing health care research and delivery as priorities in their organizational missions.[44]

Medical science is still a long way from eradicating hearing loss. Many adults who have lost some or all of their hearing are eagerly waiting for that day. Until that time comes, once you have a hearing loss, all you can do is manage it. Except for a minority of cases, hearing loss is permanent and chronic—and often progressive. This book can help you focus your efforts on adopting practices to thrive and to prevent or stave off further progression of your impairment.

Chapter Overview

The chapters in *Sound Sense* provide information about situations and environments common to people in the working ages. Work, day-to-day activities, health care, relationships, and even service dogs are all discussed. Plenty of tips that you can adapt to your circumstances and preferences are included.

Information is comprised of basics about online dating, buying hearing aids online, captioned Web videos, serving on a jury or testifying in court, filing a federal disability rights violation complaint, hearing dog politics, and current legislative efforts that may be useful to you. I conclude many chapters with an anecdote from my own life that shows the humorous side of hearing loss.

Chapter 1—Listen While You Work: Professional Development and Satisfaction—provides suggestions for getting a job, keeping a job, and developing a long-term career. This chapter also offers ideas for reducing stress in the workplace and establishing fulfilling professional relationships with your colleagues.

Chapter 2—Just Another Day in Auditory Paradise—concerns background noise, the bane of a hard of hearing person's existence. Listening challenges facing people with hearing loss include getting busy salespeople to face them so that they can speechread, hearing boarding announcements at airports, and listening to the play-by-play at a ballpark. These obstacles can seem insurmountable at times, but they are manageable. This chapter includes a wide variety of listening situations, along with ways to prepare for them in advance and to prevent many problems from happening at all.

Chapter 3—Getting a Hearing Aid or a Cochlear Implant, Demystified—provides step-by-step guidance on what to expect and what to do when you decide to get a hearing aid or a cochlear implant. This chapter includes information about insurance coverage, VA benefits, tips for saving money, and getting the best care.

Chapter 4—Sweat, Pump, Recharge, and Glow: Keeping Your Body Fit, Your Mind at Ease, and Your Ears Happy—focuses on the importance of working out and nurturing your body and spirit, even after a long day of listening. Caring for yourself will make your life healthier and your heart lighter, and this chapter contains ideas for setting up a realistic fitness program and de-stressing, along with ways to make the most of your extraordinary senses of sight, smell, touch, and taste. Be sure to try the recipe for decadent chocolate truffles at the end of the chapter!

Chapter 5—To Your Health—concerns the emotional and physical effects of hearing loss. In the elderly, hearing loss has long been associated with conditions including depression, reduced self-worth, and lowered functional capacity.[45] Adults in the working-age group with hearing loss also report dealing with several debilitating—and expensive—conditions much more often than people with excellent or good hearing. People who wear hearing aids sometimes have lower rates of these conditions than people with hearing loss who do not wear hearing aids, and the potential cost savings to the individual and to the overall health care system are substantial. Institutional investments in more widespread hearing aid use may foster massive savings to heath care providers while improving the health of affected patients. This chapter discusses these issues in detail, along with strategies for communicating with health care providers when you have a hearing loss.

Chapter 6—When Silence Isn't Golden: The Hearing Health Care Backstory—is for anyone who has ever wondered why health insurance policies seldom pay for hearing aids or offer such a small benefit. A (very brief) history of hearing aid dispensing and hearing health care politics shows many of the problems in the hearing health care delivery system. The status quo in policy contributes to many of the health inequity and quality of life problems seen in national health data with respect to hearing loss. How should hearing health delivery change to better serve patients? This chapter provides information so that people with hearing loss will be better equipped to choose a hearing health care provider who will give them the best care.

Chapter 7—Going to the Dogs: The Low-Tech Advantage in a High-Tech World—provides information about hearing service dogs, also called hearing ear dogs, signal dogs, or just hearing dogs. These animals are specially trained to alert their guardians to sounds including doorbells and knocks, telephones, and smoke alarms. This chapter details how hearing dogs work and how they are trained with their human partners, what differentiates hearing dogs from other service animals, laws pertaining to service animal access in public places, who should partner with a hearing dog, and how life changes with one of these remarkable canines at one's side.

Chapter 8—Learning for a Lifetime: Continuing Education and Career Growth—concerns reasonable accommodations for students with hearing loss. Note-takers, assistive amplification, and real-time captioning are commonly used to help students. This chapter focuses on how to get necessary accommodations and how to succeed in both coursework and on a bustling campus—whether taking a single class or pursuing a full degree program.

Chapter 9—Relationships: The Ecstasy Without the Agony—provides information about dating and socializing for someone with a hearing loss. Romantic relationships bring up not just communication issues but intimacy matters as well. Hearing aids can squawk with embarrassing feedback when people hug, for instance, and they are also not worn in bed. Simple displays of affection become potential relationship minefields. This chapter addresses these and related areas and offers ways to not just maintain but strengthen and enrich the degree of closeness in any relationship, from family members to significant others.

Conclusion—My Utopia—details my dream for an improved hearing health care delivery system.

Knowing about the resources available and having insight into "the why behind the what" in the world of hearing loss can empower you to make important decisions about your hearing health, overall health care, and professional and personal relationships. I hope this book helps you reach your goals.

Sound Sense

1

Listen While You Work: Professional Development and Satisfaction

WORK IS CLOSELY tied to a person's sense of self-worth, and a hearing loss can exacerbate any preexisting issues with self-esteem. As shown in figure 11, working-age people with trouble hearing report feeling worthless more often than people with excellent or good hearing, regardless of whether or not they are working. Within the group of people ages 18–66 who are working for pay, 6 percent of people with better hearing felt worthless at least a little of the time in the month before participating in the National Health Interview Survey. Twice that percentage—12 percent—of people with a little trouble hearing, and 13 percent of people with moderate or a lot of trouble hearing, felt worthless despite working for pay.

Not working for pay is associated with much higher rates of feeling worthless among people with all hearing abilities. Among those with excellent or good hearing and who are not working, 15 percent felt worthless at some point in the month prior to the survey, while 28 percent of people with a little trouble hearing and 33 percent—almost one in three—with moderate or a lot of trouble hearing felt worthless.

While a cause-and-effect relationship between not working and feeling worthless should not be assumed, research suggests that professionals with hearing loss are a driven bunch, doing what it takes to stay in the workforce and remain competitive despite

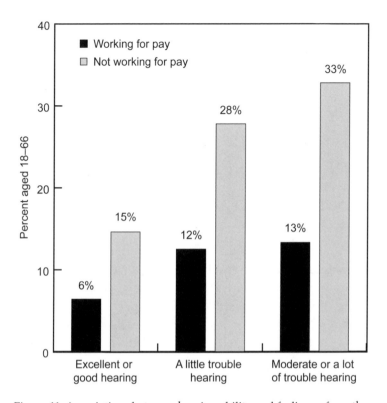

Figure 11. Associations between hearing ability and feelings of worth-lessness among working and nonworking people ages 18–66, United States, 2008. *Refused to answer, not ascertained, and don't know responses excluded.*

communication obstacles that make their jobs more challenging. Common problems include hearing on the phone, advancing in listening-intensive careers such as being a lawyer, and participating in meetings.[1]

Managing a hearing loss at work takes work, but the costs of not managing a hearing loss include reduced personal income and lower retirement savings for individuals, and lower Social Security contributions for society as a whole. Deriving fulfillment from work when you are not able to socialize or have basic communications with your colleagues becomes difficult. While disability laws mandate that an employer provides reasonable accommodations to an employee with a disability, few human resources departments are staffed with knowledgeable accessibility specialists. You may need to be proactive to get assistive technology or other solutions, or to gracefully and effectively handle employer noncompliance with the Americans with Disabilities Act (ADA) and other applicable laws.

Aside from employer-provided accommodations, there are several ways you can make your job site more hospitable and conducive to doing your best work. This chapter presents several strategies for getting a job, keeping a job, and excelling on the job, with examples and supplemental resources. Take charge of your career and don't let your hearing loss stop you!

Getting a Job

What are some good jobs for people with hearing loss? Consider your learning and working style as well as your skills before embarking on a job search. Are you an auditory learner and worker who remembers everything that she hears (not implausible for someone who used to hear better) or more of a visual person who never forgets what he sees, or do you have a strong kinesthetic nature that thrives on demonstration-based or physical tasks?

Many people are combinations of these three basic types, and finding work that exploits your natural strengths in a setting compatible with your hearing loss will make work seem less like, well, work. For example, data analysis is "hearing-lite," but if you can't stand to sit and stare at a computer most of the day, you can soon get frustrated and burn out.

If you enjoy talking and social interaction, you will likely find a job that allows you to work a lot with other people satisfying, as long as you have the amplification that you need, and relatively background-noise-free surroundings. Marketing and advertising, customer service, human resources, and supervisory work where you can lead a team are a few possible career paths. More visual people will probably excel in jobs that rely more on sight, such as photography and videography, architecture, computer game programming, and landscape design. People who love to move may consider dancing and choreography, baking, construction, and facilities management, among lots of other active jobs.

You should consider your job interests, your skill sets, and your willingness to add to your professional toolbox through continuing education or on-the-job professional development, as well as your long-term career goals. The labor force, while tight, still has a lot of options, ranging from traditional 40-hour-a-week positions to telecommuting and job-sharing positions that offer flexible work schedules.

The U.S. Department of Labor's Bureau of Labor Statistics *Occupational Outlook Handbook* gives overviews of hundreds of occupations, with information including the nuts-and-bolts of each job, working conditions, pay, and necessary training (refer to appendix B for a link to the online version of the *Handbook*). Several good books that you can find in your local library offer personality inventories and job-skills assessments; use the information that you glean from your reading and the exercises in these texts to help you narrow down your career choices. Remember that no "perfect" job exists, but with some planning (and a little luck), you can land one that is pretty close to your ideal.

After you've decided on the career paths that you would like to pursue, here are ways to get that all-important first interview.

- Networking—letting people you know that you are looking for work—is one of the best ways to get job leads. Your relatives, friends, and current or former coworkers will know about your hearing loss and are more likely to keep in mind your needs than a recruiter who may have never seen you before. Other good sources for unadvertised openings are alumni associations and social and volunteer organizations in which you participate. When you ask people to keep you in mind for job listings that they come across, let them know that you'll return the favor.
- Temporary agencies have a lot of temp-to-regular jobs, and if you are willing to start at a company on this basis you may find it to be the start of a long-term position.

- Vocational Rehabilitation (VR) centers provide job training, job counseling, placement assistance, and a host of other employment-related services to people with disabilities. Both the Department of Veterans Affairs and the Department of Education offer VR services in each U.S. state and territory to eligible applicants. Links to informational VR Web pages can be found in appendix B.

- Be careful when using online résumé posting services on job hunting Web sites, even if the companies are well known. Unscrupulous recruiters or hackers may gain access to your information without your knowledge. It is more prudent to use these Web sites as job search tools and then apply to individual postings. Never include your Social Security number, your driver's license number, credit card account numbers, or other sensitive data in a résumé, cover letter, or interview. No reputable company will ask for these specifics.

- Be cautious about giving out too much information on social networking sites. If you have a profile on one or more of them and are looking for a job, post a short paragraph describing your ideal position. Don't post your résumé, but instead give it out only to people who have a bona fide interest in helping you find work or advance your career. Keep a list of the people to whom you have given your résumé.

- Tailor your résumé to each position. Since there are about as many acceptable forms of résumés as there are job openings, it is worth spending some time looking at examples. Appendix B contains suggestions for two good books on résumé writing. A hearing loss is no excuse for sloppiness—do not expect a recruiter or a hiring manager to lower her standards for you. Make this first impression flawless and market your assets in order to be competitive from the start.

- Should you disclose your hearing loss in a cover letter? If using the phone is difficult for you, let a prospective employer know about your hearing loss in the cover letter that you send with your résumé. The cover letter should be just one page and include your most significant achievements relevant to the position for which you are applying, a sentence or two about why you are interested in the company, and your desire to set up an interview. Be sure to mention your confidence in your ability to be an asset to the employer. At the end of the letter you can mention your hearing loss and ask the employer to contact you by e-mail instead of by phone. Alternative forms of communication are reasonable accommodations for a prospective employer, and a hiring manager or recruiter should be willing and able to make them upon request.

- Should you disclose your hearing dog? There is no need to mention your hearing dog until you get to the interview stage. It is legal for you to bring your service dog to an interview, but as a courtesy, when a hiring manager schedules your face-to-face meeting, be sure to tell him or her that you have a service dog. If allergies are a concern for anyone on the job site, the hiring manager will appreciate the advance notice.

- When you have an opportunity to ask questions about the company during an interview, ask about the employer's procedure for requesting reasonable accommodations (a section on types of accommodations follows) so that you know your responsibilities for obtaining what you need to perform your duties. Employers committed to including people with disabilities will have this material available. Approaching them in the spirit of cooperation, while focusing on your assets as an employee, will get your new career off to a flying start.

- After the interview, send a paper thank you note to each person you met, including anyone who helped to arrange your meeting.

Keeping a Job

Once you have accepted a job offer (congratulations!), be sure to formally request any necessary accommodations before your start date. Many human resources employees, despite their good intentions, automatically assume that "disability" is synonymous with a mobility impairment, so you may need to educate staffers about resources available for people with hearing loss. Phone amplifiers, FM or infrared loop listening systems for large rooms, real-time captioning, and preferential seating are common ways to make hearing better at work viable. You can offer to get information to your new human resources department about specific devices, but be flexible about this approach because some employers prefer to use their own sources. Most, though, will appreciate whatever details you can get to them.

All businesses, whether small or large, for-profit or not-for-profit, are required to comply with the ADA. If you encounter resistance to your accommodations requests, speak to the designated compliance officer in your company. If you work for a small business, talk to the owner if there is no identified employee responsible for compliance.

Should you need to file a complaint for noncompliance, start with the U.S. Department of Justice. Most complaints will be directed to the Equal Employment Opportunity Commission (EEOC), but the type of employer—such as a private firm versus an educational institution—will determine the agency responsible for processing a complaint. See the Department of Justice link in appendix B for more information. Be aware that filing a complaint can be a lengthy and stressful process, but it is sometimes necessary. An employer cannot retaliate against you if you do file a complaint.

An Overview of Frequently Used Workplace Accommodations

Phone amplifiers come in two basic types—strap-on models that fit over the receiver and built-in models within the telephones themselves. Most amplifiers have adjustable volume controls, and by law these phones must be compatible with telecoil-equipped hearing aids. (The telecoil is the component in most hearing aids that works in conjunction with telephone and assistive device technology to amplify sound while making it clearer.) The amount and quality of amplification varies from brand to brand and from model to model, and it is a good idea to try out a few different amplifiers at a store such as RadioShack to find the right model for you.

FM and infrared loop systems are amplification systems that work in both large and small meeting rooms and halls, but are more common in the former. The primary speaker wears a micro-phone, and each person with a hearing loss wears a headset or a small receiver (some hearing aids can have receivers directly attached to them) that amplifies the speaker's voice directly into the hearing aids or cochlear implant speech processor. FM and infrared listening systems are also used in concert halls, movie theaters, and courtrooms.

Microphones and receivers are often battery-operated, and the venue is responsible for making sure that the system works. If pos-sible, arrange with the venue to test the system a week before you will need it. Sometimes batteries will be dead or connecting cables and wires will be tangled or lost, and the management will need to order replacements from a supplier. If you go to a performance and the listening system is not working, request a refund for your tickets from the manager. Getting your money back will not erase the disappointment, but at least you won't lose the ticket price.

Real-time captioning allows a hard of hearing worker to more easily follow multiple speakers. A captioner—similar to a court reporter—will set up a keyboard and type in all dialogue as it is spoken (in real time), which appears on a monitor in front of the employee. In essence, the worker will "see" the spoken words and be able to participate in the group exchange.

Sometimes, the captioner can e-mail a transcript of the meeting to the worker for later review. While one of the most expensive accommodations, captioning is the most useful when many speak-ers are participating in a meeting or when a few people are talking from distant points in a room, which makes speechreading nearly impossible. (Speechreading is understanding what people say by both reading their lips and getting information from facial expres-sions, body language, and the context of the situation.)

Front row or preferential seating in meetings and presentations is one of the easiest accommodations to arrange. Sitting as close to the speaker as possible enables speechreading and allows you to quickly get the presenter's attention if you need something repeated. Preferential seating is used with captioning and ampli-fication systems as well as on its own, depending on the situation.

If you are unsure of your needs, the EEOC has a superb online resource that describes various types of assistive devices and other reasonable accommodations, along with examples of situations when each might be useful in a work environment. You can find the Web site in appendix B.

If you are on assignment for a temporary agency, remember that the agency is your employer and is responsible for arranging necessary accommodations. The agency may choose to approach your assigned company to see if the firm has equipment on-site, but it is up to the temp service to respond to your requests. You are obligated to follow the procedures of the temp agency when seeking accommodations for your hearing loss.

As an example, shortly after I finished college I registered with a temp agency and explained my hearing loss at my first interview (my hearing dog was with me when I took my skill assessment tests, so everything was out in the open from the get-go). The placement representative who gave me assignments told me to let her know what I needed at each job site, and she was very responsive to my requests. She coordinated assistive amplification with my assigned company, and everything worked out well. The lesson: Don't be afraid to ask for what you need to do your job.

Accommodations also go beyond the assistive technology necessary for you to perform your tasks. The building in which you work should have emergency signaling that is accessible to someone with a hearing loss, such as strobe light smoke alarms. You should also receive written evacuation instructions to supplement any verbal material. A quiet work location—away from copiers and heavy foot traffic—can make a huge difference in your productivity, and is a straightforward accommodation that most employers can arrange before your start date.

Additional Tips to Help Make Your Workdays More Fruitful and Less Stressful

- Let your coworkers know how best to communicate with you. If you have a cube or an office, you can arrange your desk so that you are facing the entrance to your workspace. You can also ask your colleagues to flash your office light on and off a couple of times, or let them know that it is fine to tap you on your shoulder to get your attention.

- Change your answering machine or voice mail recording to ask callers to speak slowly and to repeat any phone numbers that they leave. You can also give your e-mail address in your greeting—be sure to spell it out—or suggest that people communicate with you by e-mail or text messages instead of voice mail.

- Whenever possible, schedule meetings and appointments for early in the day, so that you can listen when your ears are rested.

- Keep extra hearing aid or speech processor batteries in your desk. If you use a phone amplifier that uses batteries, keep extras of that battery size on hand as well.

- Test assistive equipment a few minutes before the start of a group meeting, so that you have time to change your seat or move the microphone without interrupting the presentation. When a guest speaker is scheduled, try to e-mail her or him ahead of time to explain that you will be using an assistive device and that she or he will need to wear a clip-on microphone. Some speakers may think that you are recording their words; if they express this concern to you, assure them that the device is for amplification only, not for recording. Ask the presenter to repeat questions posed by the audience, because you might not be able to hear them (you will probably have to remind the speaker during the address). Most lecturers and meeting planners are amenable to helping you get the most out of talks.

- Arrange with the meeting facilitator to reserve a seat for you in the front row to enable your speechreading. Sitting with your back to open windows and closing drapes or blinds where feasible will make it easier to see a speaker. Request an advance copy of the agenda or other handouts if they are available, so that you can read the material ahead of time and have an understanding of the context of the presentation.

- Don't pass up the chance to go to company parties. While it can be tempting to skip the festivities because they can be loud, instead of not going, offer to help organize the next bash and suggest to the party planners that they designate a quiet zone; lots of people with good hearing appreciate taking a breather from loud merrymaking too. Weather permitting, hold events outdoors and do not limit yourself to summer picnics—snowperson-making contests and fall harvest fairs can be good chances to get to know your coworkers outside of the office in a relaxed and fun setting.

Service Dogs at Work

If you have a hearing service dog, have a place close to you in your workspace for him so that he easily can alert you to the phone or a knock on your door. Keep a water bowl, some training treats, and a couple of toys handy, and always have poop bags available for breaks. Keeping some extra dog food in your office can come in handy if you sometimes work past dinnertime.

Your colleagues may need to be educated about etiquette toward a service dog and reminded once in a while that your dog is working and not to be distracted. If you want to dedicate some break time where humans can say hello, be consistent about playtime during work hours, for your dog's sake above all else. You may find that some of your coworkers may try to encourage your dog to break out of "work mode." If that happens, take your dog away from them immediately. Then, talk to them about the importance of knowing that your dog provides an important service to you and that interruptions can damage that relationship.

In an extreme situation, laws in all fifty states and the District of Columbia prohibit interference with a hearing service dog on duty, and you can notify the police if someone prevents your dog from performing his duties or poses a threat to her. Do not expect a supervisor to intervene in such a situation; taking care of your dog is your responsibility, not your boss's.

Excelling at Your Job

You have countless opportunities to make a name for yourself while helping your employer build its name and reputation through excellent teamwork. Some ideas follow, but brainstorm on your own and with your coworkers for more ways to contribute to your company's overall mission while developing your career.

- Offer to help improve employee morale by organizing a diversity committee to embrace the uniqueness of all colleagues. Activities can include holding a craft fair or featuring employees on the company Intranet (for instance, everyone can contribute a paragraph about how his or her background enriches the workplace). Or, offer to put together a company cookbook where employees can submit their favorite recipes and the personal stories behind them. Sales of the book can fund a corporate contribution to a charity.
- Take advantage of offers of tuition reimbursement for professional development classes and seminars. Talk to your manager about courses that will help you the most and that interest you, and follow the company's policy about documentation for your continuing education. Most firms will require proof of payment and a transcript or other official grade report that show that you satisfactorily completed the course.
- Suggest to the manager of your benefits department that your company's health plan offers hearing health benefits if it doesn't already.
- Check in with your supervisor monthly, or as often as necessary, to fill in any communication gaps that you may have missed during meetings or conferences. Do not make excuses for your hearing loss; instead, show that you are committed to fostering the effective communication necessary to get the job done. Use these meetings to go over your long-range career goals; they will show your boss that you want to continue to be a high-quality employee over the long-term, enable both of you to map out your career plans over several years, and help you decide on concrete steps to take to achieve your objectives.
- Let your supervisor know right away if something is not working for you, and suggest an alternative. If a meeting room has bad lighting, for instance, you can suggest a different

meeting room, brighter light bulbs, or real-time captioning. Most managers recognize the importance of their staffs to their success, and they want to do the right thing. When your managers do not know what to do to accommodate workers with hearing loss, show them the way, and everyone will benefit.

Supply and Demand of Workplace Drivel: A (Tongue-in-Cheek) Case Study

One day a couple of years ago, Bogie (my hearing dog) and I had an extra-early day because we had to catch a train into the San Francisco Bay Area for a meeting with a client. I spend a lot of time mucking around with data—it is in fact what people pay me to do—and having a "quiet" profession makes life on my ears that much less onerous. Occasionally I have conferences and phone calls, but in the last decade or so e-mail has eclipsed the need for a lot of face-to-face contact, which reduces long sessions of chatter that can wear out my ears in a hurry. I am used to arranging my life around listening situations, alternating meetings and socializing with auditory downtime.

On that morning I put my hearing aids in at the last possible moment, right before Bogie and I left for the train station, just to give myself a little more quiet before my meeting. My hearing aids at the time were powerful little digital buggers that made conversational speech sound as loud as the cheering at a rock concert to someone with normal hearing. It's great to be able to hear so much speech, but the amplification also makes simple pleasures such as munching crispy and crunchy toast sound like an earthquake rumbling in my head. I even choose my breakfast breads with their noise factors in mind. Untoasted bagels? No problem. Fresh croissants and scones? Terrific. Rice cakes? No way. Today was going to start with a long ride on a crowded commuter train, and that called for a scone with blackberry jam. The buttery pastry and sweet fruit spread placated my ears and buoyed my spirit. I was good to go.

The client with whom I met—I'll call him Marcus—tends to drive my ears a little nuts. Some people talk too much. Marcus, however, has raised the bar on incessant yakking; he will not, under hardly any circumstances short of coma, quiet down. I have reminded him that I bill by the hour and even that hasn't curtailed his chatter. Marcus has noble intentions, but his discussions with me tend to be monologues that wander all over the map.

Now, for those readers who know me, seeing me take issue with a person's talkativeness may raise as many eyebrows as would hearing a socialite complain about her credit lines. Give me a quarter, and I'll happily prattle on for another three minutes. As my hearing loss has progressed, I have noticed an inverse relationship between my ears and my capacity to gab: The worse my hearing gets, the more I talk. When I was in first grade, I never said a word. By the time I was in college, my professors would glance impatiently at their watches whenever I raised my hand in class.

But Marcus can out-talk me, hands down. On this day he had several ten-minute orations (I thought of them as warm-ups to the main event), and when he reached his full performance level, he talked nonstop for thirty-seven minutes and twenty seconds about absolutely nothing meaningful or relevant from what my ears and speechreading could discern. I call the phenomenon that afflicts Marcus "Speech Momentum." People (often those in a position of authority, like some bosses and politicians) who need to hear themselves talk will just not be able to stop, rather like what happens if you bicycle down a hill while pedaling as fast as you can, only find out at the bottom that your brakes don't work. The only way to end the run is to crash.

Marcus was oblivious to my glazed eyes and the yawns that I didn't bother to politely stifle after his droning hit the half hour mark. I was starting to get a headache, and I need my eyes to "hear" more than a lot of people, you know? Bogie was looking at me with his soft brown eyes pleading for respite, and when I could offer none, I gave him an organic veggie dog biscuit—one of his favorites—to appease him for another few minutes. He turned up his nose at the treat; no goodies were going to make up for this auditory onslaught. He sighed deeply, and plopped his head down on the carpet. This was not good. When a golden retriever doesn't want to eat, something is very wrong.

Marcus droned on, "and then I thought that what we should do is consider the ramifications of the potential lasting effects of the studies that we ought to pursue in anticipation of possible revisions of previous versions of our inquiries that may reveal additional comprehensive avenues for marketing exploitation that our competitors may or may not have addressed as they have been utilizing further investigations of their own to capitalize on unexplored segmentation."

Ah, he wanted to get a leg up on the competition. Okay, time for the bicycle to crash. I loosened the cap on my water bottle and then dropped the bottle on the carpet while jumping in feigned surprise, letting out a startled cry of, "Oh no! I'm so sorry!"

"So we should scrutinize and document . . . what?" Marcus asked, abruptly breaking off from his last tangent. (His last word is usually my line, by the way.) Speech Momentum appeared to be skidding on a road of broken glass, heading for road rash. I was putting some billable time at risk, I realized, but I was trying to get the job done, and I couldn't do anything with our lopsided communications already in a state of entropy.

I apologized again for spilling the water, and I mopped it up with the towel that I keep under Bogie's water bowl. It was silent for a few delightful moments; Marcus knows that I can't speechread when I am looking at the floor. With the water bottle situation under control, I knew that I needed to prevent Marcus from opening the verbal floodgates again.

"Marcus," I said sternly as I stood up with the dripping wet towel in my hands, "Please tell me, using no more than ten words, what you need to know. I cannot help you otherwise." I could see his mind and his mouth struggling with each other. "Pithy" was not in Marcus's vocabulary.

He opened his mouth, closed it, and then finally opened it again and said, "I need to know what our competitors are working on now." Well, that's eleven words, but he was trying, so I cut him some slack.

"Thank you," I said. "That is helpful. I will put together a research outline and e-mail it to you by tomorrow, okay?" He nodded but still looked like he was trying to get his head around the concept of expressing his needs so economically. (I am guessing that he reads a lot of postmodern philosophy. Out loud.) We said our good-byes, and Bogie and I both heaved deep sighs of relief on the elevator down to the lobby. I leaned my head—it was still pounding—back on the elevator wall and pressed the wet towel against my forehead. Most of the morning had evaporated—the time seemed like much longer than a morning—and my ears were beyond saturated with listening.

Bogie and I caught the last train home. The cars were nearly empty and blissfully quiet. Passengers disembarking earlier had taken their background noise with them. I found a row of seats that was not littered with the day's worth of coffee cups and newspapers, and I shrugged off my backpack before flinging myself down on the aisle seat and whooshing an utterly exhausted sigh.

My thoughts wandered to my experiences in the labor force, which started more than thirty years ago. I have had different jobs with different listening demands, but none as quirky as Marcus's. Early in my hearing loss years, before listening got really difficult, I worked for years as a pizzeria hostess and then as a snack bar attendant. When my hearing loss progressed to the point that hearing in those more chatter-heavy settings was too hard to navigate, I became a chocolate truffle maker (see chapter 4 for a recipe). After I got my hearing aids and was able to obtain more training, I went into bookkeeping and project management and then into my current research and demography work.

Now I spend most of my time in quiet surroundings, which works out well for me. I use assistive listening devices, real-time captioning, and preferential seating to enable me to hear in meetings, and both my hearing aid and cochlear implant have telecoils that allow me to use the phone a little bit, although hearing on the phone is always a challenge. E-mail has made my professional life much easier and more effective than it was fifteen years or so ago, and I prefer that mode of communication.

I am lucky—and I know it—that technology has enabled me to continue working in my chosen field and that most people with whom I interact are empathetic, even when they exhaust me, like Marcus.

Bogie nudged my arm. I looked around for the source of his alert, but saw none. I guess the train whistle must have blown, because we started to pull out of the station.

"Bogie," I said, nodding toward my feet, "Sit." He sat. I gave him a treat. "Down," I said. He dropped his front paws all the way down. I gave him another treat. "Stay," I said. He stayed. I scratched his ears, which perked up as the train picked up steam. Ah, the power of one-word sentences. Marcus can learn a few things from them. But. So. Can. I.

2

Just Another Day in Auditory Paradise

BEING A CONFIDENT self-advocate is important whether or not you have a hearing loss. Having special needs because of your hearing makes it even more essential that you are able to take care of yourself in whatever circumstances your life brings. No one can navigate your life as well as you can.

Without question, living with a hearing loss in a hearing world is hard. Your hearing loss informs every decision you make on some level—where to have lunch, how to get flight information at an airport, and how to communicate with the produce manager at your local supermarket. Dealing with daily hurdles such as these can be so frustrating that it may be tempting to become a hermit!

It can also be exhausting. At times, it can feel as if you are living a life and a half, constantly anticipating auditory challenges and thinking ahead to possible solutions. One big positive to keep in mind, though, is that almost all listening is based on context and expectation. When you go to the library, for instance, you can reasonably expect the librarian to ask for your library card when you go to the counter to check out your books. Generally, situations like these carry little stress and are straightforward.

But when you take the context out of the communications equation, you can wind up with a talking curve ball that can flummox you and make your blood pressure skyrocket. Imagine, for example, going to a gift-wrap kiosk at the mall and hearing the person who works there ask you if you wear your hearing aids at the gym. It would likely take the worker several repeated tries before you understand the unexpected comments. Both of you would wind up irritated. Communications chasms like these can make everyone involved regret making small talk.

I call these episodes "van Gogh Moments," or VGMs, for Vincent van Gogh, the 19th-century Dutch painter who cut off part of his left ear. While I have not gotten to that point, often, after being unable to understand what someone is saying, I want to go to the kitchen, throw my hearing aid and cochlear implant processor into the garbage disposal, and flip the switch. (Yes, common sense has always kicked in, and I am happy to report that my ear hardware is still intact.) I have a hearing aid in one ear, a cochlear implant speech processor in my other ear, and a hearing service dog at my side; try being inconspicuous when you're a walking mixture of lopsided high-tech bionics and low-tech dog fur. When I factor in the stares, gawks, or pointing fingers, it becomes easy to see how one too many insensitive comments can trigger a VGM.

The good news is that VGMs pass, and afterward they offer valuable lessons in the importance of being patient with myself and others, and of being nimble in my thinking about how to manage routine happenings. Don't let one sour event turn a day into a chain of negativity. Move on and move forward.

This chapter contains lots of strategies for managing daily listening needs using a three-pronged approach. First, reduce noise exposure whenever possible; second, use available equipment and devices to hear better at home and at social events; and third, try new strategies to hear and live better just about everywhere and monitor how your efforts work for you.

A Noisy World

Noise exposure is a widespread cause of hearing loss among the working-age population (refer to figures 8 and 9 in the introduction). The trappings of modern life, including exposure to loud music, create a racket that can assault our ears around the clock. How noisy is a typical day? The chart in table 2 shows the loudness of common sounds expressed in decibels. A value of zero equates to silence, conversational speech rates about 60 decibels,

Table 2. Decibel chart of everyday sounds

Sound	Decibels
Refrigerator	45
Clothes dryer	60
Washing machine	65
Vacuum cleaner	70
Electric shaver	85
Hand drill	100
Car horn or siren	120

Source: U.S. Department of Health and Human Services, National Institute on Deafness and Other Communication Disorders, Noise: Keeping It Down at Home, http://noisyplanet.nidcd.nih.gov/staticresources/materials/Parent Tipsheet_KeepDownatHome.pdf (accessed November 2, 2009).

and sounds that are at least 85 decibels can cause noise-induced hearing loss over time.[1]

The encouraging news is that you can prevent hearing loss or its progression due to noise exposure. What are some good ways to reduce noise exposure at home? Staying away from loud sounds is the best prevention, but is not always a viable tactic. Wearing good-quality ear plugs (available at most drug stores) is an effective way to prevent noise-induced hearing loss when you cannot avoid being around it. If you use hearing aids or a cochlear implant, turn off your devices when you operate noisy equipment, such as the garbage disposal or the vacuum. Run your washer and dryer when you are away from home on errands, and consider using a push mower instead of a gas-powered mower. Dual-pane or laminated windows, although pricey investments in home improvement, will buffer noise as well as outside temperatures.

Think of quieter alternatives for noisy situations. For example, instead of meeting friends at a pizzeria on a busy night, have a "make your own pizza" party at home. If you enjoy baseball, going to a minor league game instead of a major league ballpark will be both quieter and less expensive. When weather permits, go for a hike or take a walk outside instead of mall walking where background noise tends to be high. Actor Larry Hagman practices "a rule of silence" on Sundays,[2] which is a novel way to give your ears some much-needed rest.

Assistive Equipment to Use at Home

Take advantage of technology, such as using captions on your television while turning the volume down or off. People in the working-age group with hearing loss most often use closed-captioning and television headsets. Among people in this group who reported using any assistive listening device in the 2007 National Health Interview Survey, 66 percent benefited from captioning or amplified headsets.[3]

Captioning

Captions on a screen display in words the audio part of a television program or commercial. Captions also describe sound effects, such as a doorbell ringing or background music, by using words or icons such as musical notes so people who rely on captions can "read" all of the audio information in a program. Captions are being used more and more by people without hearing loss—many gyms, sports bars, and loud restaurants that have television monitors keep the caption function turned on—so that everyone can benefit from the technology.

Since July 1, 1993, new televisions with a diagonal measurement of greater than 13 inches must be equipped with internal closed-caption decoders.[4] An external captioning decoder can be connected to a television not equipped with an internal decoder, but these older models are increasingly difficult to find. Whether a decoder is internal or external, captions look the same on the screen. Digital television service providers are also required to make captioned programming available, although digital televisions may not show captions if the television is not configured correctly at home, or if the digital television service provider has systematic problems that block captions.[5]

The Federal Communications Commission (FCC) oversees compliance with captioning regulations and requires that most, though not all, programming be captioned. Exceptions include nonfederally funded programming less than ten minutes long (such as commercials), and programs for which captioning would present a hardship to the producers as documented by petition to the FCC.[6] Exemptions are not easy to get; the FCC is serious about making as much programming as possible accessible to people with hearing loss.

The costs of captioning are reasonable. According to the National Captioning Institute, approximately 200 captioning companies charge from $2 to $10 per minute for their services, which is not a lot of money considering the multimillion-dollar budgets of most network shows. Depending on the complexity of the project, captioning accuracy for live television runs about 98 percent, and pre-recorded programs have captions that are close to 100 percent correct. Technology also exists to caption Internet videos, and several software packages allow do-it-yourself online captioning.[7] Links to these resources can be found in appendix B.

Closed captioning can influence an individual's consumer and political decisions. Many people who rely on captions make it a practice only to patronize businesses that caption their commercials or vote only for political candidates who caption their advertising. If you decide to not buy a product or service or to not vote for a candidate based upon the absence of captioning, send an e-mail to the business's or candidate's Web page to let them know why you are not supporting their missions.

Amplified Telephones

Amplified telephones are another commonly used form of assistive technology. Over one-third—37 percent—of the working-age population with a hearing loss uses an amplified phone.[8] These devices have come a long way in the past several years, and they have better sound quality whether or not you use a hearing aid with a telecoil. Some phones can even be used with cochlear implant speech processors, although even in the best of circumstances using the phone with a cochlear implant remains difficult. The amplifiers are generally built into the phones, and many have adjustable volume settings.

Most states have programs that provide free amplified phones and related equipment to residents with a hearing loss, regardless of financial need. Typically, the state provides a form to complete with identifying information, and your doctor or audiologist signs the form verifying your hearing loss. You can try out the phones available before choosing one to take home. The equipment remains the property of the state and must be returned if you move.

The Telecommunications Equipment Distribution Program Association contains a directory of state equipment programs on its Web site (included in appendix B). Several private firms also manufacture and sell amplified phones. As with state-provided equipment, always try out the equipment to make sure that it will work for you.

Other Technology

Other forms of assistive technology include strobe light smoke alarms, FM and infrared listening devices that amplify speakers from several feet away (often used in lecture halls or courtrooms), and alarm clocks that vibrate under your pillow instead of ringing next to your bed. Despite the widespread availability and afford-ability of most assistive technology, just 4 percent of people ages 18–66 with difficulty hearing reported using *any* form of these devices in 2007.[9] Put another way, more than twenty million addi-tional working-age adults could benefit from assistive listening equipment other than hearing aids and cochlear implants.

Everyday Strategies for Dealing with Hearing Loss

Numerous additional ways exist to deal with hearing obstacles throughout the day, and most of them are easy to apply to your life. The following tips can help you while running errands, enjoy-ing holidays and special events, traveling, or just having fun.

Two Golden Rules to Help You Hear Better Everywhere, Every Day:

1. **Make your needs known.** Speaking up for yourself is your responsibility and no one else's. Do not assume that other people can read your mind. Your most important strategy is proactivity. Plan ahead and anticipate your needs, and then communicate them to people with whom you interact. Be clear, concise, and polite.

2. **Rely on common sense.** The most important accommodation that people can give to you is their common sense. Tell everyone to feel welcome asking you how she or he can help you hear better. Do not let other people assume that they know what is best for you.

Tips for Hearing Better While Taking Care of Everyday Tasks

- Think safety first. Install a peephole in your front door if you cannot hear a response to "Who is it?" when someone knocks on your door or rings the doorbell. If hearing those alerts is difficult, check into visual equipment, such as a lamp that flashes when there is a knock or a ring. Appendix B contains sources for these devices. Also, recent research indicates that strobe light smoke alarms are less effective than low-frequency audio alarms at waking up people with mild to moderate hearing loss.[10] Check into the most recent technology before purchasing or upgrading your home safety systems—you may need more than one kind of smoke alarm or alerting apparatus to stay safe.

- This tip offered in chapter 1 bears repeating: keep spare hearing aid batteries in several places—your wallet or purse, your desk at work, your backpack, your laptop case, and your gym bag are all convenient places to stash portable power. Keep extra batteries for your assistive devices at home and at work, too. Few events are more annoying than running out of batteries when you really need to hear something or someone!

- Remember your civic duty. Having a hearing loss will not get you out of jury duty. If you receive a summons for jury service, contact the court right away to let the administrator know about your need for either an assistive listening device or real-time captioning. As a courtesy, if you have a hearing service dog, it is a good idea to give the administrator a heads-up about your canine partner as well.

- Speak up about loud music. If a restaurant has blaring music, ask the manager to turn it down if it is interfering with your conversation. Sit with your back to windows or lamps; speechreading is much easier without a bright light shining in your face.
- Try to dine at off-peak times to reduce the number of voices your hearing aids or cochlear implant need to process. Choose out-of-the-way tables at restaurants that are carpeted to help buffer background noise. Restaurants with outdoor seating offer another option that can be easier on your ears than establishments where sound bounces off of every surface.
- Sit at round tables in restaurants. Round tables can make group communication easier than rectangular seating. Along the same lines, the fixed seating and uncarpeted floors common in fast-food restaurants can make hearing and speechreading challenging.
- Shop at smaller stores when possible. They can be quieter than big department stores.
- Avoid noisy service bays when talking to your mechanic. Talk to the service manager away from noisy areas and get estimates and repair details in writing, to help prevent misunderstanding the work that needs to be done on your vehicle.

Tips for Hearing During the Holidays and Special Events

- At the Thanksgiving table, use low centerpieces and good lighting to make speechreading easier. Sit where you can comfortably speechread—have lighting above and behind you, not in front of you—and remind everyone to face you when they talk to you. Ears tired from all of the chatter and clatter? Take a break and go for a tranquil walk. The exercise can help your fitness, too.
- Thinking of staying in on New Year's Eve to watch the Times Square ball drop from home? Send an e-mail to the broadcast network or your local station in mid-December to confirm that

the program will be closed-captioned. FCC regulations require captioning for these television specials, but sometimes— especially for one-time-only events—local broadcasters need to be reminded of this requirement.

- Fourth of July fireworks are fantastic visual displays, but the pops can wreak havoc on your ears. Turn off your hearing aids or speech processor before the show starts.
- Weddings and funerals can require extra-special sensitivity. You need to be able to hear at these events, but the wedding hosts or the family of the deceased are seldom in a position to help you with accommodations. Religious organizations are excluded from complying with Americans with Disabilities Act accessibility requirements, but some houses of worship do have listening systems. If time permits, inquire about availability before the service. If a wedding or a memorial takes place in a public venue, check with the facility manager to see what assistive devices are available.
- If you have a hearing service dog, always ask your wedding hosts if it is permissible to bring your dog to the festivities. Your dog is allowed access to public places by law, but if the wedding is in a private home, or if members of the wedding party are allergic to dogs regardless of where the wedding takes place, the right thing to do is to leave your dog at home as a courtesy to the hosts.
- Several hours of loud music and festivities may also be hard on your dog, so keep his or her needs in mind as well. At a funeral or a memorial service, keep your dog off the grass in a graveyard.

Tips for Hearing Better While Traveling

- When you travel by plane, let the airline know that you are hard of hearing when you make your reservation. Often you can note your hearing status on the online reservation form. If you can't hear flight announcements and no visual message board exists in the boarding area, ask the airline representative at the departure gate to notify you when it is time to board or if there are any delays. You can also ask to preboard the plane. Once you're on the plane, let a flight attendant know how he or she can best communicate with you.

- Take all of your hearing aid accessories in your carry-on baggage and be prepared to have airport security personnel check through everything. A cochlear implant may trigger a response from a metal detector, so let a security guard know ahead of time that you have the device. Federal Aviation Administration regulations allow the use of hearing aids and cochlear implants in flight.[11]

- When you plan your next vacation, e-mail individual attractions and the convention and visitors bureaus of the cities you will be visiting to find out about services for people with hearing loss. Many public venues, such as baseball and football stadiums and theme parks, have facilities hard-wired for telecoil-equipped hearing aids or offer captioned informational films.

- If you will be staying in a hotel and need an amplified phone, a closed-captioned television, a strobe light smoke alarm, or any other assistive technology in your room, e-mail the property before you make a reservation to ask about the availability of these accommodations. Most hotels and motels, including franchises of larger chains, have Web sites with e-mail addresses that go directly to an individual facility. Include in your e-mail a specific list of what you need and your travel dates. Ask for an e-mail confirmation from a manager of what equipment is available and in working order—often, properties have assistive devices, but they are broken, connection cords are missing, or batteries are dead. Also, request the name of a contact person at the property in case problems arise when you arrive.

- Hotels are required by the Americans with Disabilities Act to provide reasonable accommodations for a disability, but they do not have to offer a specific brand of amplifier, for example. If you do not receive a response to your e-mail query within a few days, or if the reply indicates that what you need is not available, you may want to consider staying somewhere else.

Few hotels or motels are able to purchase new equipment or repair broken devices on short notice. If you do contact another hotel, be sure to mention that its nonresponsive competitor could not serve your needs. That news will almost guarantee that you will be a properly pampered guest at the second property you contact.

- Be prepared for a common misconception among hotel staff about disabilities in general. Identifying yourself as having any type of disability when you make a reservation may get you accommodations equipped for someone with a mobility impairment, such as a room with a wheelchair-compatible roll-in shower. If you would like a standard room, ask for one and get a written confirmation with your reservation.

- If you have a hearing service dog, be sure to mention that your canine companion will accompany you. All fifty states and the District of Columbia require that properties with a "no pets" policy permit hearing dogs access to their facilities, including on-site restaurants or breakfast rooms.

- After your stay, send a note to the hotel manager with any compliments or suggestions for improvement. If you had an exceptionally good experience, you may want to post a summary of it on a Web-based travel review site so that other people with hearing loss can learn about a good place to stay away from home.

Tips to Help You Have More Fun

- Newer technology for enjoying movies includes Rear Window Captioning, which displays captions on a small monitor right at your seat. Not all theaters offer Rear Window Captioning, but dozens of theaters in the mainland United States are already equipped with this accommodation. Appendix B contains a link to an online directory of venues with this technology.

- Think small when wine tasting—boutique wineries are usually a lot quieter than the big name tasting rooms.

- Encourage your local restaurant reviewers to include noise ratings of local eateries in their write-ups. Regardless of hearing ability, many people like to dine in relative peace and quiet and will appreciate having information on how loud a restaurant is before making a reservation.

- If you like water sports, make sure to bring along a plastic zip-top bag to store your hearing aids while you are in the pool or ocean. Keep tabs on your companions and never go into the water alone.
- If you enjoy going to concerts or if you play or sing in a band, turn your hearing aids or cochlear implant speech processor down or off when using amplification. One nonprofit organization, Hearing Education and Awareness for Rockers (H.E.A.R.), targets its outreach to musicians of all ages because the problem of hearing loss has not been well-acknowledged by many people in this population segment (see appendix B for a link to the H.E.A.R. Web site).

My Life Is a Battery

Before Halloween every year our local fire department sends out a reminder to change any smoke alarm batteries. The notice I received got me thinking about how dependent I am on auxiliary power, which is a rather scary thought since I pride myself on being independent. I scribbled—for my own information at first—the following "Top Ten List of Equipment and Geegaws that I Use that Run on Batteries." When I finished, I contemplated buying stock in a power-cell manufacturing company and keeping the shares until I retire. In the meantime, I'll keep on stocking up on batteries when they go on sale—a good idea for anyone who relies on auxiliary devices!

1a. Hearing aids—where would I be without these digital miracles? My power-junkie aid churns through a button battery every week or so, much to the joy of the electronics department manager at my local discount store.
1b. Cochlear implants—since getting my implant two years ago, I have turned into a zinc-air battery madwoman. Most hearing aid and cochlear implant disposable batteries are

the zinc-air variety, and my speech processor drains three of these big-kahuna-size 675 hearing aid batteries every three days, if I am lucky. I also use rechargeable batteries, each of which provides power for about ten hours. (I love to show the charger to airport security whenever I fly—it looks like something out of a *Mission Impossible* movie, complete with a couple of buttons that look as if they may cause the whole thing to self-destruct.)

2. Assistive listening devices (ALDs)—I've got both a single-speaker FM system that I use for conferences and the multispeaker tabletop model that works in small group settings. The manufacturer says that the AA batteries used in these ALDs should last three hundred hours each, but the manufacturer must be misinformed. I consider myself lucky if the juice lasts two weeks. In theory these ALDs also run on rechargeable batteries, but in practice, the rechargeable batteries that came with the ALDs have never been able to hold much of a charge. Last I heard—in 1998—the manufacturer was "making progress" on correcting the defect.

3. Smoke alarms, carbon monoxide detectors, and strobe lights—if, heaven forbid, there is ever a fire in my house, the place will start flashing like a 1970s pinball arcade that would make Elton John proud. We must go through more 9-volt backup batteries in our house than babies go through diapers.

4. A strobe light door-knock alert—this puppy eats up two AAA batteries every couple of weeks. You can't see it flash its strobe alert unless you're standing right next to the door, but since it looks cool and is a conversation piece among people with normal hearing, it stays up and winks every once in a while to remind us of its presence.

5. Phone amplifiers—I both adore and despise these things. While they let me have voice communications, they also suck the life out of AAA batteries every few days. At least their low-battery indicators let me know when they're gasping for their last breath of life.

6a. Vibrotactile alarm clock—to supplement a hearing dog, these alarm clocks go under a pillow and shake, rattle, and roll when the alarm goes off, thanks to several batteries that power the clock itself, the backlight, and the alarm mechanism. Fifty years from now if my complexion is glowing gamma green, I'll know why. Try one if you ever want feel the magic of genuinely scrambled brains under bed-head first thing in the morning.

6b. Bed-shaker alarm clock—for heavy sleepers, or for non-Californians who want to experience what an earthquake feels like, these devices run on several size D batteries that trigger the slumber-shattering megatemblors and are calibrated to get someone out of your bed—and occasionally out of the rest of your life too—in a hurry.

7. Wireless doorbell—I use this doodad to practice signal training with my hearing dog. It runs on some odd-size battery that I can never remember, and the battery always seems to go kaput when I am practicing the signals without wearing my hearing aids. I don't know that the doorbell chime isn't going off until my beloved dog gives me an exasperated stare. No bell equals no treat, which isn't the way the world is supposed to work when you're a hearing dog. Canine priorities are so simple; I should learn from them.

8. M4-rated cell phones—one of the most recent technological marvels, they allow much better hearing on cell phones now than in the past, especially for people who have telecoil-equipped hearing aids. The batteries are rechargeable but expensive to replace if you are inclined—as I am—to drop and break small expensive special-order electronic things. I inherited the klutz gene from my mother's DNA pool; no wonder everyone on that branch of the family tree is a technophobe.

9. Laptop computer—while not specific to people with hearing loss, of course, the battery was just recalled and is on my mind as my too-warm wrists rest on the battery port. The recall mentioned something about the battery overheating and catching fire. (Better the computer than my hearing aids,

you know? Talk about having a bad hair day.) I changed the smoke alarm batteries, just in case.

10. The car—ah, the car. After being awakened by a vibrating alarm clock and a hyperactive hearing dog, I put in my hearing aids and called the computer store on my amplified phone to confirm that the laptop replacement batteries were in stock. All of my power systems were fully operational until I tried to start the car and found out that *that* battery was dead.

I find lessons and mixed metaphors here that I am still sorting out. Am I making progress? I'll let you know in about ten years.

3

Getting a Hearing Aid or a Cochlear Implant, Demystified

Buying a hearing aid, or getting a cochlear implant, requires taking a huge step forward. When you make the decision to get amplification, myriad other choices follow—the type of aid or implant, where to make the purchase, and payment arrangements are three of the most important. This chapter describes the types of amplification available and who can benefit from them, a step-by-step overview of the purchase process, and a summary of available hearing health care benefits. While most health plans will pay for cochlear implants, the majority of hearing aids are out of pocket expenses. Progress in third-party payment for these devices is being made, albeit slowly. What to expect with your new amplification follows, and the chapter concludes with tips for getting better hearing health care and how to save money while doing it.

Types of Amplification Available

While no hearing aid or auditory implant can restore hearing, today's sophisticated technologies enable people with hearing loss to reap substantial benefits from amplification, feedback control, and comfort improvements in hearing aids that are far superior to the devices available just twenty years ago. Descriptions of conventional hearing aids, surgically implanted hearing devices, and cochlear implants, along with advantages and disadvantages of each type, follow.

Conventional hearing aids are the kind of aids that you put on and take off each day. Manufacturers make them in three basic types:

1. In-the-canal and completely-in-the-canal aids, which are the smallest and the least visible;
2. In-the-ear aids, which sit in the part of the ear that you can see; and
3. Behind-the-ear aids, which rest on top of the ear and are secured by a custom earmold that fits in your outer ear. Newer "open-fit" hearing aids are variations of the behind-the-ear models, so-called because no earmold sits in the outer ear or ear canal.

To process sound, conventional hearing aids use either analog or digital technology that is customized for an individual patient to provide improved sound perception and speech discrimination, and reduced feedback. Most people with sensorineural hearing loss—which is caused by damage to the ear nerves and is the most common type of loss—can benefit from hearing aids. Out-of-pocket costs for hearing aids can be substantial and include the purchase price of the aids (less any available health insurance benefits for the devices), repairs, follow-up visits with an audiologist or hearing aid dispenser, optional extended warranty coverage, and batteries.

You can order disposable hearing aids online. These products cannot be customized to a person's individual hearing loss, and they are designed for people with mild to moderate hearing loss. Because disposable aids are not custom-fit, a person who uses them may experience whistling and feedback. Despite these drawbacks, disposable hearing aids are much less expensive than traditional hearing aids, and they might be worth trying as a way to get an idea of how amplification can improve quality of life. The volume can be adjusted, and no battery purchases are required; when the battery dies after about three months of use, the user replaces the entire hearing aid.

Surgically implanted hearing devices are also grouped into three categories:

1. Bone-anchored hearing aids (Baha), suitable for people with conductive hearing loss (due to damage to the outer or middle ear), mixed hearing loss (both conductive and sensorineural), or deafness in one ear only;
2. Newer middle-ear implants, designed for people with moderate to severe sensorineural hearing loss; and
3. Auditory brainstem implants, which can help patients who have become deaf due to auditory nerve damage.

Surgically implanted hearing aid systems are not completely invisible. The processors that transmit sound to the implants are worn externally. These devices run on battery power, and battery life varies by the type of implant system. Candidacy for surgically implanted devices varies, but in general, patients who qualify for the surgical procedures do not benefit from conventional hearing aids. Health insurance usually covers the cost of the operation for most surgically implanted hearing devices, and Medicare covers bone-anchored hearing aids and auditory brainstem implants. Copayments and deductibles are the patient's responsibility.

Cochlear implants are very sophisticated, multipart electronic devices. They are designed for people with severe to profound hearing losses, and candidates for implantation derive no appreciable benefit from hearing aids. A patient will need to spend considerable time learning how to hear with an implant in the months following surgery because the sound is completely manufactured (in contrast to hearing aids, which amplify sound that a patient's ear can still perceive). Sounds usually do not sound natural at first. People who have lost their hearing after learning to speak can adapt very well to the cochlear implant, but people born clinically deaf can also experience a marked benefit. Some babies born without hearing are implanted when they are a little over one year old. While most people receive an implant in one ear only—generally, the ear with the worse hearing—binaural implantation is becoming more common as research has documented the advantages of having an implant in each ear. Batteries that power cochlear implants are usually attached to the external speech processor and can be rechargeable or disposable. Battery life ranges from about ten hours (for rechargeables) to about three days (for disposables). Both private insurance and Medicare pay for cochlear implants, less copayments and deductibles.

Electric acoustic stimulation (EAS) implants combine hearing aid and cochlear implant technologies to benefit people who have severe to profound hearing loss in the middle and high frequencies (which include most consonants used in speech, birds singing, and related pitches), but less than severe hearing loss in the low frequencies (which include sounds such as vowels and a refrigerator humming). Research suggests that EAS implants can benefit people with this kind of partial deafness, but the procedure carries the risks of surgery, and because EAS implants are just beginning to be used in the United States, health insurance plans may not cover the operation.

Choosing the right device depends on the type and severity of hearing loss, and personal preferences. Most people with hearing loss can benefit from conventional hearing aids, and these devices carry no surgical risks. When necessary, however, and when a person with a hearing loss is comfortable with having an operation and committing to postsurgical aural rehabilitation, the surgically placed devices can offer tremendous improvement in quality of life and self-reliance.

The Hearing Aid Purchase Process

As shown in figure 12, there are five steps to getting a hearing aid.

1. Realize and accept that you need amplification. Once you have cleared this hurdle, the process can be a rewarding and healthy experience. One way to start thinking about whether or not you are ready for hearing aids is to make a list of all of the situations and environments that are challenging for you without amplification. Some examples include watching television, hearing groups at work, driving in traffic, using the phone, attending large lecture classes, and

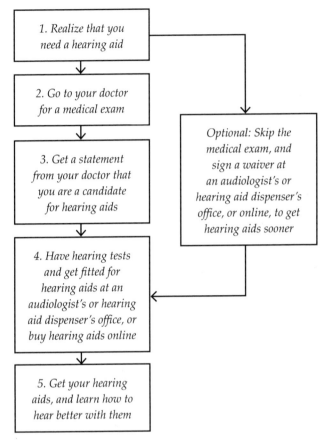

Figure 12. The hearing aid purchase process, step-by-step

power-walking around the neighborhood. If you are having trouble engaging with the world or find that you are unable to live your life the way you want or need to, give hearing aids a try. Most states mandate trial periods—usually thirty days—for these devices, so if they truly do not work out for you after a few weeks, you can return them for a refund (often less a fitting or other administrative fee).

2. Get a medical examination within six months of your hearing aid purchase.

You do not need a prescription to buy a hearing aid, but you do need to have your ears checked by a physician—ideally an ear, nose, and throat specialist—before purchasing a hearing aid to determine the cause of your hearing loss. Your doctor can determine if your hearing loss is due to a reason that requires medical attention or if hearing aids are a viable alternative for you.

Audiologists and hearing aid dispensers (referred to in this chapter as "practitioners" or "dispensers") are not qualified to diagnose or treat some causes of hearing loss—Meniere's disease or ear tumors, for example. Although a hearing loss for these reasons is less common than sensorineural hearing loss caused by noise or aging (also called "presbycusis"), not ruling out these serious conditions can let a potentially life-threatening condition go undiagnosed.

3. Get a statement from your doctor that you are a candidate for hearing aids. If your doctor determines that a hearing aid can work for you, you will receive a physician's statement confirming that hearing aids are suitable for your hearing loss. You can take that document to the dispenser of your choice. No standard form for this statement exists; your doctor can choose how to give you the information. Some physicians write letters while others have their own forms that they complete and give to you.

Since the possibility exists that a person may have a hearing loss due to a serious medical condition, it is not a good idea to bypass the doctor's exam. However, you are legally allowed to do so by signing a "waiver" of the medical exam. Dispensers will provide a waiver form to you that you must sign and that they must keep on file for three years.[1] While online merchants have electronic versions of waivers available on their Web sites, think carefully before bypassing a physician's checkup.

Consider the possibility that companies or practitioners (whether online or bricks-and-mortar establishments) who make it easy for you to sign a waiver may be more interested in selling you a product than they are in helping you improve your health. If anyone tries to push you into signing a waiver, run—don't walk—away, and go somewhere more reputable. Anyone who sells a hearing aid has to be licensed by the state in which he or she is doing business, so you can check with your state's Department of Audiology or Department of Hearing Aid Dispensing Office for the license status of a practitioner. File a complaint if necessary with the same department.

4. Go to a dispenser for testing and hearing aid fitting. The practitioner will administer several hearing tests in the office to determine the extent and nature of your hearing loss and to help determine the hearing aids that are likely to work best for you. The tests are not invasive or painful. You will listen to various tones to determine how loud they are before you perceive them, and the dispenser will conduct some other ear functioning assessments and speech discrimination evaluations at the same time.

   It is not unusual to have different hearing in each ear, and hearing aids can be set to accommodate for the disparities so that your hearing will be pretty well balanced when the aids are customized to your ears. You may also need just one hearing aid, depending upon the results of the evaluation. If your tests show that you do need two, having both will make a big difference in your ability to hear, but getting one is still better than getting none.

   Be sure to bring your list of situations where you most often experience difficulty hearing to your appointment; that information will also help the dispenser narrow down the best hearing aids for your lifestyle. After you order your hearing aids, it may take about two weeks for the manufacturer to deliver them to your dispenser. Expect to feel excited and a little impatient!

5. Start to hear with your new hearing aids. When your aids arrive, you will need to go back to your dispenser to pick them up and have them programmed (if you are getting digital aids). This process may take a few hours, and you will probably have to go back a couple of times for programming adjustments. During the programming you will wear the aids while your dispenser adjusts the settings on a computer. You can report back on how things sound and changes can be made on the spot.

Dispensers must provide everyone who purchases a hearing aid with information on the use and care of the aid, as well as an address to which a hearing aid may be sent for repairs. New hearing aids should come with at least a one-year warranty from the manufacturer. Some dispensers also offer extended coverage (at your expense) for repairs after the initial warranty period expires. These policies can also include coverage for the loss or theft of your aids. If you think that a high risk of either of those events happening exists, or if the cost of one average out-of-warranty repair is the same or greater price than the cost of the extended warranty plan, it is a good idea to get this extra protection.

Ask as many questions as you need to feel fully informed about your purchase. You should also get a couple of packages of batteries (if your aids don't have rechargeable batteries) included with your aids. Some dispensers offer "battery clubs," but these may not save you money. Discount stores and some online merchants usually have better prices, and Sunday newspapers often have coupons for brand-name batteries.

When you walk out of the office wearing your aids for the first time, expect to be startled by how noisy things sound. The rumbling of a bus or the clatter of dropping your keys on the floor can make you jump. You will probably be hearing some sounds for the first time in a long time, such as water running and birds chirping.

Your dispenser may recommend that at first you wear your hearing aids for just a few hours a day, but the sooner you are wearing them whenever you are awake, the faster you will adapt to them. Practice listening on the phone—call someone whose voice you know well—and go into familiar stores and restaurants to get used to hearing in them. Be patient with yourself, and take your time adjusting to the hearing world. Take care of your hearing aids, and they should last at least five years.

Choosing What You Need, and Knowing What You'll Get

In general, the smaller the aid, the less amplification it will provide, so bigger aids (most often the traditional behind-the-ear models) are usually best for people with severe hearing losses.

Smaller, less visible hearing aids can also be more expensive than larger hearing aids. Earmolds and hearing aids come in different colors, so you can match your hair or skin tone or go funky and get fluorescent green.

Based upon your hearing loss and your daily listening needs, your dispenser will discuss other features with you, such as the processing type (analog or digital), built-in telecoils that allow you to use the phone and some assistive devices, and multiple microphones. Most hearing aids can be set with several different "programs" that allow you to adjust the settings with the touch of a button to compensate for various situations during the day, such as a noisy store or watching television at home.

Next, your practitioner will show you several different models and brands. Most offices sell only a few brands; some audiology clinics based in research hospitals or hearing institutes offer a wider selection than a smaller practice. Do not make your choice at your first visit; take any brochures or informational DVDs that are available and review these materials on your own. Look up the company Web sites for more details.

Hearing aid manufacturers are competitive, and most products made by companies that do business with reputable dispensers offer high-quality products. The difference in how one aid will sound compared to another is not easy to quantify; technical specifications do not translate into subjective preference. You will not know exactly how a hearing aid will sound until you try it.

After you narrow down your choices to a few models that you and your practitioner think will work, order the least expensive model from that group. Unless you are trying an open-fit hearing aid, your dispenser will make earmold impressions in the office by squeezing thick goo (usually silicone-based) into your outer ears and letting it harden for a few minutes before removing the finished impressions. The earmolds enable a custom, secure fit for your hearing aids, and your practitioner will help you decide on the best type for your hearing loss.

An external lab will use the impressions to make earmolds for behind-the-ear hearing aids or the casings for in-the-ear or in-the-canal aids. The lab will send everything to your dispenser. Earmolds sometimes do not fit correctly on the first try, and it can take a few days for any discomfort or feedback to manifest itself, so make sure to contact your practitioner if a problem occurs with how your earmolds fit. Dispensers can make some earmold modifications in their offices, but occasionally, they will have to take new impressions and send those back to the lab.

Over time, earmolds for behind-the-ear hearing aids will need to be replaced. In general, you should be able to get at least a year's use out of them. Significant weight loss or gain can change the fit of earmolds and necessitate their replacement. If you notice a sudden tightness in how your earmolds fit, or any pain or redness, you may have an ear infection and should see an ear doctor right away. The thin tubing that connects the hearing aid to the earmold also can crack, causing horrendous feedback. Many dispensers will give you spare tubing to take home, but others will require you to make an appointment for this repair.

When your hearing aids need more extensive repairs, you must take them to your dispenser. Hearing aid manufacturers will not accept direct shipments from consumers. This allows the dispenser to check the aids, and often they can handle simple repairs on-site. However, if the manufacturer has to do the job, be prepared to wait several weeks for the aids to be returned to your practitioner. Some dispensers have loaner hearing aids, and others do not. Be sure to confirm repair and loaner policies when negotiating the purchase contract. Some dispensers also offer faster turnaround times for repair if you pay for express shipping.

Payment arrangements are expected when you order your hearing aids. Usually, a dispenser will require a 50 percent deposit if your insurance does not cover the aids, but practices vary. You should get copies of the following on a signed and dated form when you order your hearing aids: the purchase agreement, including all payment terms; the receipt of a deposit; the right to cancel if the aids are not delivered within the stated timeframe; all warranties; the trial period; and the number of follow-up visits and accessories included in the purchase price. If you are paying cash, this is the time to negotiate any discounts and to make sure that those are noted on the purchase agreement. Do not accept any verbal promises—if they are not in writing, do not bank on your dispenser honoring them.

Where Can You Buy Hearing Aids?

Dispensers may have free-standing offices or operate out of a physician's practice, a hearing institute, a large medical center, or even some department or big-box retail stores. They may market their products on the Internet. Internet-only dispensers often work with multiple office-based dispensers. You can order hearing aids online, but for most models, you will still need to go to a dispenser's office for earmold impressions and hearing aid programming. Getting the best fit and programming (for digital aids) possible will increase your chances of a successful experience and reduce the likelihood of squeaky feedback.

Who Can Sell Hearing Aids?

Permissible sellers vary by state. Audiologists, hearing aid dispensers, and even physicians can sell hearing aids. All practitioners are state-licensed, and each state establishes requirements for licensure and continuing education. A blurry—and sometimes overlapping—line exists between hearing aid dispensers and audiologists. Hearing aid dispensers do not have to be audiologists to sell hearing aids, but, depending upon the state regulations, an audiologist must sometimes be licensed as a hearing aid dispenser to sell hearing aids (see chapter 6 for more details on why this policy exists).

Audiologists are licensed in every state. In some states, an audiologist can dispense hearing aids by virtue of having an audiology license only. Some states allow professional association certifications for licensure as well.[2] The sale of used hearing aids is permissible in some states; individual states regulate these transactions and who can conduct them.

Hearing Health Care Financing Today

Effective January 1, 2009, the Federal Employees Health Benefits Program (FEHBP) implemented hearing aid coverage for current and retired federal employees and their dependents. Benefits vary but are typically limited to about $1,000 per ear and are available once every three to five years.[3] At the state level, Rhode Island is the only state that mandates that third-party insurance plans offer hearing aid benefits for everyone, although fourteen other states (Colorado, Connecticut, Delaware, Kentucky, Louisiana, Maine, Maryland, Minnesota, Missouri, New Jersey, New Mexico, Oklahoma, Oregon, and Wisconsin) have hearing aid benefit requirements for children.[4] (As an interesting trivia note, Rhode Island was home to Aime Forand, the U.S. representative who in 1959 introduced the bill that evolved into Medicare six years later.)

Some audiologists and hearing aid dispensers offer financing options, either on their own or through a third-party administrator. Many also accept credit cards, and some have other discount programs. One chain of hearing aid offices in the Seattle, Washington, area offers a discount through a private automobile club. Such discounts may not sit well with everyone; can you imagine a cardiologist, for example, offering an auto club discount for an electrocardiogram?

If you are comfortable doing business this way, and the dispenser is highly regarded, discount programs can offer savings. Be wary if a practitioner tries to up-sell your planned purchase after finding out that you qualify for a discount, and try to compare prices at a few dispensers before making your decision.

The Hearing Aid Tax Credit

Over the past several years, lawmakers have proposed legislation to offer taxpayers a credit for hearing aid purchases, in lieu of mandates for third-party coverage. No previous bill has become law. The current bills (H.R. 1646 and S. 1019) allow for a $500 credit per hearing aid once in a five-year period; the Senate version covers people of all ages, and the House version limits the tax credit to hearing aids for adults at least 55 years old and for the dependents of taxpayers. Both bills are currently in committee.

While this credit may sound wonderful, be sure to read the fine print. If you itemize your deductions on your federal income tax return, you will not be able to deduct the cost of your hearing aids if you take the tax credit—you can do one or the other, but not both. If the tax savings from deducting your hearing aid purchase will be greater than the value of the hearing aid tax credit, then the credit will be worthless. Also, for those who are eligible, $500 every five years boils down to less than fifty-five cents per day for both ears, which will barely cover the cost of batteries for many people. Before giving your support to this proposed legislation, consider advocating instead for mandatory hearing aid benefits in third-party health insurance policies and think about who will really benefit from the current bills.

Many of the bill's supporters are hearing aid manufacturers and organizations of hearing health care professionals, with an obvious interest in the marketing power of a tax credit. Insurance coverage requires hearing aid dispensers and audiologists to complete a lot of paperwork, but the documentation burden for a tax credit is on the individual taxpayer.

The Patient Protection and Affordable Care Act, signed into law by President Obama on March 23, 2010, does not address hearing health care. Hearing aids or other hearing devices are not included in the list of essential health benefits mandated by the legislation,[5] and audiology services are not brought up anywhere in the entire document (though specific services such as dental care and vision care are mentioned). Whether the failure to mandate hearing health care benefits was a deliberate omission or an accidental oversight on the part of legislators remains unclear. While coverage for hearing aids may be added to essential health benefits down the road, it is a safe bet that achieving mandated federal coverage for hearing aids for everyone covered by the act will require many years of Herculean effort.

Hearing Aids and the Department of Veterans Affairs

The Department of Veterans Affairs (VA) provides more hearing aids to Americans than any other entity, and its role as a hearing aid dispenser continues to grow. In fiscal years 2007 and 2008, the VA dispensed one out of every seven hearing aids sold in the United States, and its share of the market increased to one in six hearing aids (17 percent) during the first half of the 2009 fiscal year. The VA has such massive purchasing power that it pays an average of only $355 per hearing aid to its suppliers.[6] Compare this amount to the average retail price of $1,676 per hearing aid,[7] and you can see how economies of scale benefit the consumer.

While many recipients of hearing aids from the VA are World War II veterans and other retired military personnel, the VA also provides hearing devices to service personnel as young as 18 years old. Veterans who qualify for hearing aids from the VA can receive upgraded hearing aids from the agency when equipment is no longer adequate; some current recipients are more than 90 years old.[8]

Table 3 shows the number of hearing aids the VA has dispensed to its entire service population since 2005, rounded to the nearest 1,000.

An individual veteran's disability category determines out-of-pocket costs or copayments for hearing aids from the VA. "Service-connected" hearing loss—in other words, a hearing

Table 3. Hearing aids dispensed by the Department of Veterans Affairs, fiscal years 2005–08

Year	Number of hearing aids dispensed	Rate of increase from previous year (%)
2005	309,000	n/a
2006	312,000	1
2007	349,000	11
2008	382,000	9

Source: U.S. Department of Veterans Affairs, Denver Acquisition and Logistics Center, Veterans Health Information Systems and Technology Architecture data.

loss caused directly by military service—does not require any patient payment. "Nonservice-connected" hearing loss will trigger a copayment between $50 and $150, unless the patient has other service-related disabilities that result in a disability rating (as determined by the VA) of at least 50 percent.[9] Even if a copayment is required, the amount is a real bargain compared to prices charged by private dispensers.

The VA provides hearing aid batteries on request; patients who have hearing aids that are approved in the VA system—including hearing aids purchased outside the VA—can order batteries at no charge by phone, e-mail, regular mail, or online.[10] Assistive devices, including amplified telephones, vibrating alarm clocks, and FM listening systems, are available through VA audiology departments.[11] While the VA does have a program in place to train and place guide dogs for people who have visual impairments, as well as service dogs for people with mobility impairments, hearing dogs are not available through this agency.[12]

If you are a veteran with hearing loss, check with your nearest VA outpatient clinic to find out about hearing health care services for which you may be eligible at little or no cost. These services can offer tremendous benefit.

Tips for Better Hearing Health Care

You can be proactive about getting the necessary care for your hearing loss, and do so in efficient and cost-effective ways. Several suggestions follow.

- Remember—you're the customer when shopping for new hearing aids. Don't be afraid to ask hearing aid dispensers about their policies regarding extra costs after your initial purchase, especially repair fees, reprogramming charges, and replacement earmolds that may surprise you. If you don't get clear answers, go to another dispenser.
- Many local drug stores offer buy-one-get-one-free specials on hearing aid batteries throughout the year, so stock up when these buying opportunities come up.

- Itemize deductions on your federal tax return. Hearing aids and their batteries, mileage to and from your audiologist, and hearing service dog training and care are acceptable medical expenses according to the Internal Revenue Service (IRS). IRS Publication 502, *Medical and Dental Expenses*, contains more information—check with a tax expert for guidance on your individual tax situation. Refer to appendix B for a link to this publication.
- Store your "electronic ears" in a dehumidifier container at night or whenever you're not wearing them. Warm weather can wreak havoc on your hearing aids or speech processor because sweat, mist from lawn sprinklers, and humidity can damage the devices.
- Make sure to "re-bake" your hearing aid or cochlear implant processor dehumidifier drying unit during the rainy season, in order to help keep your devices in good shape. Always follow the manufacturer's directions for reactivating the moisture-absorbing material. While you can microwave the pellets in some types of drying units, never nuke the metal versions.
- Remember to dispose of used batteries in accordance with your local waste regulations.
- Order everything at the same time and you shouldn't have to pay for a second set of impressions. A dispenser can use the same impressions for your hearing aid earmolds and swimming earplugs. You can also request that your impressions be saved or returned to you for future use, but not all practitioners will agree to do this.
- Ask your audiologist and doctor about new technology and noise-prevention strategies. The technology improves continuously but all too frequently once your audiologist has sold you a pair of hearing aids, discussion of assistive technology and aural guidance stops. Check the Web site for your hearing aid or device manufacturer occasionally to find out more about the capabilities of your equipment and the proper care of it.
- Find others who are willing to provide service beyond the sale if your health care providers don't have time to answer

your questions. Hearing aid manufacturers often have referral services on their Web sites. If you do change providers, send a letter to your old provider explaining why you made the switch. Stick to the facts and make no apology for taking the best care of yourself. When it comes to your health, you need to vote with your feet, your wallet, and your pen. And, most of all, use a clear, confident, and proud voice.

Getting a Cochlear Implant

When your hearing loss is severe enough, you can have an audiologist and cochlear implant surgeon evaluate your hearing to determine if you are a candidate for an implant. The hearing tests and medical evaluations will take about half a day and will include several hours of speech discrimination and hearing tests, a physical examination, a discussion with your doctor or other health care providers about your expectations for the cochlear implant procedure, and often a cochlear magnetic resonance imaging (MRI) examination. Ask as many questions as you need to during these appointments.

Because the cochlear implant contains a magnet, after the surgery you will be able to have MRI diagnostics only under very controlled conditions that may require additional surgery to remove the implant magnet prior to the MRI test. Your surgeon can tell you the limitations of each type of implant with respect to MRIs and other medical treatments. (Some surgically implanted hearing aids also contain a magnet.)

If you are a candidate for an implant in one or both ears, you will have to decide on the brand of implant that you want. There are three manufacturers of Food and Drug Administration (FDA)-approved cochlear implants—Advanced Bionics, Cochlear Americas, and MED-EL. Your surgery center may offer implants from one, two, or all three manufacturers.

An Interesting Caveat

No health care practitioner will recommend one brand of implant over another, because of the potential for ethical violations. As one

example, Cochlear Americas and Cochlear Limited were alleged
to be in violation of the Federal Anti-Kickback Act and the Federal
Civil False Claims Act when they "made direct cash payments to
Physicians and/or paid for trips to exotic locations for Physicians
and their spouses or guests and families. The express purpose of
such payments are and were to encourage Physicians to direct hospitals, as purchasing agents, to purchase Cochlear Implant Systems."
Additional instances of payments of tens of thousands of dollars to
physicians or their clinics as incentives to buy additional Cochlear
products were also cited in this civil action.[13] On June 9, 2010, the
U.S. Department of Justice announced that Cochlear Americas
would pay $880,000 to the U.S. government to settle the lawsuit,
which was filed in 2004 by a whistleblower, Brenda March.[14]

If you are getting an implant, a decision for a life-altering device
that will be surgically installed in your head, you will have to
make the decision without medical input from your implant team
about a particular brand. Doctors and audiologists will answer
questions about the specific attributes of a model—such as the
available colors of a speech processor—but it is highly unlikely
that they will be willing to express a preference for one device
over another because of the ethical boundaries that they may
violate by doing so. We are laity, not hearing health care professionals, yet we are charged with making a choice that requires
substantial medical and technical expertise. It is a daunting task.

Your implant team will send you home with a stack of slick
marketing brochures and some informational DVDs produced by
the implant manufacturers. After that, it's up to you. You can—
and should—contact the manufacturers directly with questions
and use their answers to inform your decision. Ask your implant
team members to put you in touch with other implantees. You can
ask questions and discuss your concerns with people who have
"been there and done that."

Implants and the speech processors (implants are internal and
the speech processors are the parts worn over the ear, and that
you take off at night, when showering, or when swimming) have
gotten very sophisticated, and the technology will likely help
you hear far better than you can without the devices, no matter

which brand you select. Differences between brands include the range of hearing frequencies that can be amplified, the processing technologies, and the colors and styles of the external processors. Regardless of manufacturer, the implant itself is about one-and-one-half-inches long by one-inch wide, and less than one-quarter of an inch thick. It is surgically attached to the skull under the skin behind the ear. An electrode array extends down the implant, and the surgeon threads the array into the cochlea to enable stimulation of the auditory nerve. The externally worn sound processor has a microphone that transmits sound to the implant. Newer sound processors look like behind-the-ear hearing aids. A thin wire cable about four inches long extends from the processor, which is connected to a magnet about the size of a half-dollar coin. The magnet attaches to the scalp on top of the internal implant (which also contains a magnet), and as the external processor receives sound information, it passes through the wire cable and into the implant. The system does sound somewhat "Frankensteinish!"

Preparing for Cochlear Implant Surgery, and What to Expect After the Procedure

After you decide to have the procedure, you will be scheduled for surgery. Because of an increased risk of bacterial meningitis in cochlear implant users, the standard protocol at many implant centers is to administer vaccinations for this infection at least six weeks before surgery. You will also need to have presurgical laboratory tests a few days before the procedure. Your doctor and audiologist will probably meet with you again at that time and give you final instructions for surgery day. Bring a list of any remaining questions that you have about the operation or aftercare.

Also, if you are having one implant and not two, arrange for someone—typically a recovery room nurse—to keep your hearing aid during the operation so that the nurse can give it to you as soon as you wake up. Putting the aid in your nonimplanted ear will give you some sound awareness right away, which can help to orient you in what can be a very confusing environment.

When I had my implant surgery, the anesthesiologist let me wear both of my aids until right after he wheeled me into the operating room. He took them out after I was asleep, and gave them to a nurse who had them waiting for me in recovery. I couldn't use a hearing aid in my implanted ear, but having the aid in my unimplanted ear was definitely better than having no amplification as I started to regain consciousness.

You should consider bringing an oversize, button-down shirt to the hospital to wear home; you will not be able to easily pull on a t-shirt or other top with a narrower neck opening because of the protective bandages that the surgeon will apply during your operation. If you wear glasses, you will need to unscrew and remove the earpiece on the side of your head that receives the implant. Your ear will be completely covered with the bandages, and the earpiece will not fit over them. Yes, your glasses may look a little lopsided for a few weeks, but it is only temporary.

Before surgery day, stock up on groceries and prepare meals ahead of time to last for a few days. Your surgeon will let you know if there are any dietary restrictions to keep in mind. If your doctor allows it, I recommend having lots of ice cream in your favorite flavors waiting in the freezer!

The surgery takes two to three hours and is done on an outpatient or inpatient basis (mine was an outpatient procedure; I was in and out faster than same-day dry cleaning). Right before your operation, you may feel very nervous, but that's natural—getting an implant is a major life change. Right after your surgery you will probably feel like you just got off of the world's worst roller coaster.

For the first few days after your surgery, expect to feel some pain and dizziness. You may not want to eat much for a while and will likely be content to take it very easy. Some implantees find it more comfortable to sleep sitting up, propped by pillows, until the worst of the dizziness is over. As you can see in the picture on the next page, it is very easy to fall asleep this way.

If you are married or living with a partner, he or she should plan on staying with you for a few days after your surgery to help with your care needs and household tasks. If you live alone, try to arrange for a friend to stay with you, or see if you can stay with him or her until you can take care of yourself. Most doctors prohibit bending over or lifting more than a few pounds for several

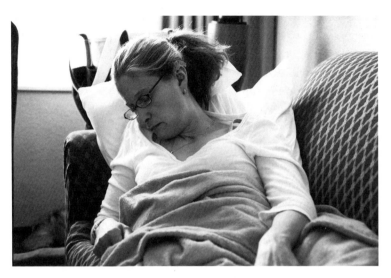

The author, doing what she did best three days after her cochlear implant surgery. Her hearing aid is in her nonimplanted ear. Note the snoozing hearing service dog in the background. Part of the Keep Sara Humble Collection. Photo credit: © 2008 John S. Batinovich. All rights reserved.

weeks, and you will not be able to drive until you are no longer dizzy. Be careful to not trip over any pets. You may not be able to see if your dog or cat is right next to you because it will be hard for you to peer all the way down while keeping your head upright. You will also not be able to shower or get your hair wet for a few days—although most patients can take baths in the meantime—since you will have to wear a protective cup over your implanted ear (or ears) during the initial healing process.

You will not be able to hear out of your implanted ear(s) for several weeks because the surgical site needs to heal before the implant is "activated." On that day, your surgeon will clear you for activation and then send you to the cochlear implant audiologist (generally in the same facility; he or she will have specialized training for cochlear implant tasks) for programming your speech processor. This process will take about half a day, and it will be tiring but also exhilarating. Expect your first sound perception to be strange and unnatural, but your brain will quickly adapt to the new auditory input.

Be sure to give your audiologist detailed descriptions of how things sound so that she or he can adjust your processor in order to make what you are hearing sound as natural as possible. Your audiologist will also give you exhaustive instructions on how to care for your equipment and show you how to insert the batteries, put all of the components together, and store the processor when not in use. When you need replacement parts, you can get them directly from the manufacturer or from your audiologist if the policy at your implant center allows for it.

Regular follow-up visits with your surgeon and implant audiologist are important, and additional programming appointments will fine-tune your processor as you get used to hearing with your newly implanted ear. Enjoy the process of hearing sounds that you haven't heard for so long! One of my favorite ways to practice listening is to play music from twenty or so years ago, so my auditory memory can help me hear the great melodies that my implant interprets in its whiz-bang, 21st-century bionic fashion.

How I Became a Bionic Bride

I had been a candidate for binaural cochlear implants for a few years before I decided to take the plunge and have the surgery in one ear. While my ears were ready, my heart was not—the surgery is not without risks, there is no assurance of success (although the likelihood is high), and part of me was still hoping for a medical miracle that would restore natural hearing through auditory cell regeneration.

But early in 2008 I got engaged, and I started thinking more about making communication in married life as easy as possible. Everyone told me that it was challenging even with good hearing! John—my intended, and now my husband—has always been understanding about my hearing loss, but it did get frustrating for both of us at times when John kept having to repeat himself, or I couldn't hear him from more than a few feet away.

A couple of months later, at my ear checkup, my hearing tests showed further decline. My audiologist and ear doctor could see how much I was struggling to have conversations with my hearing aids maxed out on their amplification capabilities, and my doctor—who has been taking care of my ears for almost twenty years—told me with kindness in his voice, "We knew that this day would come." At that point, new hearing aids would not give me any more benefit; I already had the power version of very advanced digital hearing aids that were far from obsolete, and they just weren't enough anymore. And my dream of a medical breakthrough is not likely to be realized in my lifetime. In my gut, I knew that the implant was the right step for me at that point.

I had another round of cochlear implant candidate evaluation testing, and I was definitely qualified for the procedure. When the doctors explained the advantages of the newest generation of implants, I felt encouraged and ready to move forward with scheduling the surgery. Implants and speech processors have come a long way in twenty-five years, and the current models have the capacity to create sound that is much more natural than was possible in years past. Implants can be used with future generations of the external processors, so additional surgery will not be necessary to take advantage of the advancements; reprogramming can be done without more invasive procedures.

The surgery went well, and my adaptation to bionic hearing has been very smooth and successful. At my initial activation appointment, I was able to hear my audiologist when she covered her mouth, and that had not happened in decades! That first appointment took about four hours, and when I took a break and went to the bathroom, I fully appreciated the power of the implant for the first time: When I flushed the toilet, the noise was so loud that I almost had a heart attack!

Since then, I have learned to hear in routine and unfamiliar situations. While my hearing will never be "normal" as far as my audiogram is concerned, and some listening circumstances—such as hearing on the phone—will always be challenging and fatiguing, I have enjoyed a remarkable improvement in my ability to discriminate speech and other sounds. I can usually hear John when he calls me from another room, and I can pick out more dialogue on television now (though I still rely on captioned programming).

I was surprised that many people asked me shortly after my surgery if I was planning to keep Bogie, my hearing dog. Above all else, Bogie is my canine best friend, and I would rather cut off my arms and legs than give him up. But as far as my ears are concerned, Bogie is still very much an essential assistance to me. I don't wear my speech processor at night, when I shower, or when I swim, and Bogie alerts me to sounds during those times, because I hear nothing then. My implant—despite the sensational technology—also does not give me a good sense of sound directionality, but Bogie's ears never fail to point me to the source of a voice or other auditory stimulus. And while my hearing is much better with the implant, many sounds, including a door knock, still escape me, but Bogie alerts me to those immediately.

It has been two years since my surgery, and music appreciation is what I work on the most these days. I continue to make progress in discriminating different notes and chords, and I am looking forward to advancements in speech processor development that will permit even greater music perception. For now, I smile when I recognize a once-familiar song. And on John's and my wedding day, when the wedding march played at the start of our ceremony, I was able to hear it!

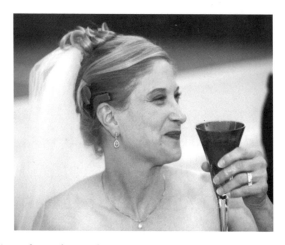

Cheers from the author on her wedding day! The "Bionic Bride's" cochlear implant speech processor is visible above her ear. Photo credit: © 2008 Joe Buissink. All rights reserved.

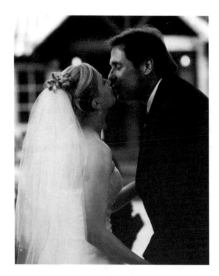

The Bionic Bride and her handsome groom, John Batinovich, celebrate being pronounced husband and wife. Photo credit: © 2008 Joe Buissink. All rights reserved.

4

Sweat, Pump, Recharge, and Glow: Keeping Your Body Fit, Your Mind at Ease, and Your Ears Happy

PEOPLE WITH A hearing loss know that stress often accompanies it. According to the National Institute of Mental Health, "Anxiety is a normal reaction to stress," and generalized anxiety tends to be chronic, manifesting itself as worry, fatigue, nausea, headaches, irritability, muscle disorders, insomnia, and other ailments that can be long lasting and require expensive treatment.[1]

Relatively common among all people in the working-age group, people with hearing loss have higher rates of anxiety relative to people with better hearing. As figure 13 shows, almost one in five people—18 percent—with excellent or good hearing has experienced generalized anxiety at some point in their lives; nearly one in three people—32 percent—with any trouble hearing has had general anxiety; and 33 percent of people with moderate or a lot of trouble hearing report having had this condition.

Exercise and Healthy Behaviors

The serious effects of anxiety and stress mean that people with hearing loss need to be aware of the symptoms, work to prevent them, and address them when they appear. Lifestyle changes such as good exercise and sleep habits are effective ways to manage stress,[2] and they can be incorporated into daily life even with a hearing loss. As noted by the Mayo Clinic, "Regular exercise can

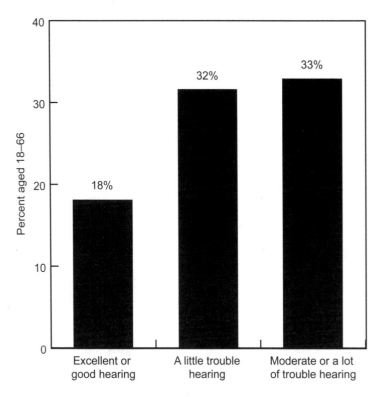

Figure 13. Generalized anxiety by hearing ability, people aged 18–66, United States, 2008. Author calculations of 2008 National Health Interview Survey data. *Refused to answer, not ascertained, and don't know responses excluded.*

increase self-confidence and lower the symptoms associated with mild depression and anxiety. This can ease your stress levels and give you a sense of command over your body and your life."[3]

This chapter contains suggestions for a healthy lifestyle and stress reduction, along with ways to maximize your compensatory senses of touch, smell, taste, and sight that can enrich your everyday experiences and further reduce stress. The chapter concludes with a recipe for one of the best stress-busters of all— chocolate truffles.

Hearing Aid Use and Healthy Lifestyle Behaviors

Working-age people who use hearing aids have higher rates of some healthy behaviors than people with hearing loss who do not use hearing aids. Figure 14 shows the differences between these populations for adequate sleep and exercise.

Among the working-age population wearing hearing aids, 51 percent engage in light or moderate exercise at least two times per week and 46 percent of the working-age population who have

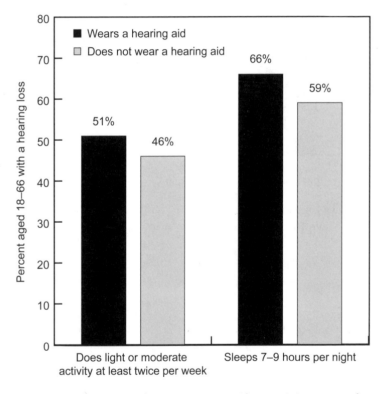

Figure 14. Differences in physical activity and hours of sleep per night among people ages 18–66 with hearing loss, by hearing aid use, United States, 2008. *Light or moderate physical activity is defined as leisure-time physical activity done for at least ten minutes, causing only light sweating or a slight to moderate increase in breathing or heart rate. Refused to answer, not ascertained, and don't know responses excluded.*

trouble hearing and do not wear hearing aids perform this level of physical activity. The hearing-aid wearing group also has a higher rate of sleeping seven to nine hours per night. Sixty-six percent get adequate sleep while 59 percent of people with hearing loss who do not wear hearing aids sleep the same number of hours.

It is possible that working-age people who wear hearing aids are more committed to a healthier lifestyle or have the time to exercise and sleep more. These findings suggest that hearing aids are associated with healthier behaviors within an individual's control. Primary care physicians may want to consider promoting more hearing aid use among their hearing impaired patients in conjunction with lifestyle changes that lower stress and improve overall quality of life.

Exercise with a Hearing Loss

With the knowledge that hearing loss often comes with stress and that exercise can mitigate its effects, it makes sense to commit to physical fitness. Certainly, exercise includes a host of other well-known benefits, including body fat reduction, increased muscle tone, and cardiovascular conditioning. Yes, working out is yet another time commitment, but if you are not exercising, give it a try (after you get your doctor's go-ahead) and see how your physical and emotional health change when you are active.

The President's Council on Physical Fitness and Sports recommends that adults get thirty minutes of exercise at least five days a week, but you can incorporate chores such as yard work and walking your dog into that allotment to reach the half-hour goal.[4] Here are some ideas to get you started and keep you motivated.

- Pick activities that you enjoy and that don't demand a lot of listening. Swimming, stationary cycling, walking, and weight training are good choices. Strive for a balance of cardiovascular training (aerobics), strength training (weights and other resistance exercises), and stretching or relaxation (such as yoga or tai chi) each week.
- Keep in mind that guided meditation tapes can be a source of stress instead of relaxation to people with hearing loss. Watch

a captioned yoga workout tape straight through without doing the routine to get the basic ideas. Then, give the poses and breathing techniques a try.

- Consider trying out home workout DVDs. Dozens are closed-captioned, and just about every type of workout is available in this medium, from kickboxing to stability ball routines. You can't beat the convenience of working out at home, and most workouts give excellent instruction so that you can exercise safely using the proper techniques. Many of these DVDs are available from online rental services or at your local library, so you can try several at low or no cost.

- Be extra-vigilant when exercising near traffic. During your walks, runs, or bicycling workouts wear fluorescent clothing with reflective tape, and make eye contact with drivers before you cross the street. Avoid working out whenever visibility is reduced, such as during heavy commute hours, at sunrise and sunset, at night, or when the weather is foggy or rainy. Carry a flashlight or wear a headlamp if you must be outside after dark.

- Don't forget that classes at gyms and fitness centers can be problematic when you have a hearing loss because you won't always—or even consistently—hear the instructions. I was almost decapitated once during a martial arts class years ago because I didn't hear the instructor shout, "Sara, roundhouse kick behind you!" until what turned out to be his fourth attempt to get me to hear him, and nobody in the room was happy. A few sweaty souls looked at me like I was from another planet. Since then, I have used the gym mostly for solo training, saving myself and scores of innocent people from injury. I do the riskier activities—anything involving kicks and punches in particular—at home.

- Keep an exercise journal with your workout progress or note your workouts on your calendar. Write down what you like doing the most, what is problematic, and how you feel after each exercise period.

- Be proud of yourself for your fitness accomplishments!

Nutrition and Hearing Loss

Good nutrition is essential no matter what your hearing status is, but when you are getting fit, eating right takes on even more importance. Your doctor or nurse practitioner can give you guidance on what you need specifically, but in general, eat balanced meals, stay away from too much junk, and drink lots of water. Try not to eat for an hour or two before your workout, but get some healthy food into your body soon after you finish an exercise session.

Is there a correlation between nutrition and hearing loss? Research is limited in this area, but scientists conducting studies reported by the National Institute on Deafness and Other Communication Disorders have discovered that some micronutrients may help prevent noise-induced hearing loss when taken before exposure to loud noises, such as concerts. Vitamin E, vitamin C, magnesium, and beta-carotene are thought to be responsible for preventing the damage.[5]

While preventing hearing loss by avoiding loud noises or by wearing ear protection are still the best ways to protect your hearing, taking advantage of new knowledge from nutritional researchers can also help enhance your life. Check with your doctor for advice before taking supplements, as they may interact with your medicines or exacerbate existing conditions.

Tips to Avoid Stress and Nurture Your Spirit

- Remove your hearing aids or speech processor before you brush or comb your hair—these devices are very easy to damage.
- Take off hearing aids and cochlear implant speech processors before using shaving cream, face cream, lotion, or makeup—all of these products can damage your equipment, necessitating costly repairs.
- When using hair gel, spray, pomade, leave-in conditioners, and related products, make sure that your hair is completely dry before you put on your hearing aids or speech processor.
- Shower or bathe at night, to prevent wet ears in the morning. You can also blow-dry your ears before putting on your hearing

aids or speech processors. Showering at night can also tempo-
rarily mask tinnitus symptoms and help you get to sleep.

- Brush your teeth with warm water at night to help you relax
  and with cold water in the morning to help get you going.
- Try using a hair clip or bobby pin to secure the coil cable of your
  cochlear implant speech processor to your hair if you wear your
  hair loose or down. People who use a cochlear implant can go
  bonkers trying to find hairstyles that won't knock off the magnet. Ponytails work well for men and women.
- Make sure any headgear fits comfortably over your hearing
  aids or speech processors. Baseball caps and bike helmets may
  need to be adjusted to feel secure and be comfortable.
- Buy clothes with your ears in mind. Zippered sweatshirts are
  more convenient than are hooded designs or other pullovers,
  and button-down shirts won't knock off ear hardware.
- Be aware of the effect that air temperature can have on your
  hearing devices. Some cochlear implant speech processors
  can malfunction or stop working when the temperature drops
  below about fifty degrees Fahrenheit (ten degrees Celsius). I
  wear a snowcap to keep my processor warm on days that are
  chilly. Otherwise, it sounds like I am trying to receive trans-
  missions from Antarctica!
- Rest on one side when taking a nap, with your hearing aid or
  speech processor worn on the other side.
- Use a blow dryer or a soft towel to dry off your ears and
  nearby scalp after your workout since sweat can affect the
  performance of a hearing aid or speech processor.
- If you swim, use caution when strapping goggles over your
  cochlear implant site—the straps should not be too tight. Brightly
  colored swimming ear plugs will keep water out of your ears and
  signal to others that you won't be able to hear them well.
- When you go to a barber or hair salon, explain to your stylist
  that you cannot wear your devices while she or he is cutting
  your hair. Get all questions answered before you take out your
  ears, especially before no-turning-back decisions like getting
  a new hair color or cutting off several inches of your tresses.

Most stylists are trained to talk to you by looking at you in the mirror, so you shouldn't have to turn your head to speechread. Have a pad of paper and a pen available for questions during your styling.

- Eliminate obvious stressors when you can—don't bother, for example, to try to listen to the sound effects in a bowl of crispy rice cereal.
- Keep a "health log" for a month. Record foods, activities, and interactions that most strongly (and weakly) affect how you feel afterward. Note how many hours you sleep and how you feel right before getting into bed and right after you wake up. See if you can find patterns in how you feel and the duration and quality of your nightly rest.

Compensatory Senses

When you have a hearing loss, you are often perched in the middle of two worlds, drawing on all of your senses to enrich and complete the parts of your life that your ears cannot fill in. You hear with your eyes—which people with normal hearing also do, of course, though they are probably not as aware of it. You can feel silence, see speech, smell fear, and taste life more acutely than a lot of people with better hearing.

John, my wonderful husband, says that I notice *everything*— nothing gets by me, especially his flaws!—and that skill can come in handy. When someone loses his or her hearing, other senses become more important. I fully appreciated how much I relied on sight and smell a few days after my cochlear implant activation. John—then my fiancé—and I went to a movie, and I saw a popcorn machine at the concession counter spilling out freshly popped kernels by the thousand.

That buttery smell hit me, but something else did, too—for the first time in about thirty years, I really *heard* the popcorn popping. All of those years, I thought that I was hearing the popping sound, but what I was really doing was remembering it. My auditory memory combined with my senses of sight and smell created a sound that wasn't there, but to me, it was powerfully real. Since then, I have been much more aware of the interaction among my senses, and the richness that the interplay gives to mundane situations when I pay attention to what everything along with my ears tells me.

The next section describes ways to celebrate life using your other senses during everyday experiences and how to use ordinary things around the house to help make each day extraordinary. Give your whole being a renaissance with these ideas for rejuvenating and energizing your everyday life and your home, sense by sense.

Touch

- After a long day of listening, pamper yourself from head to toe. Take out your hearing aids, soak a cotton ball in warm water, and squeeze out the excess. Swab the damp ball around your outer ears and let the warmth melt your stresses away. Then, divert your attention from your ears to your toes with a relaxing footbath. Aromatic flower petals or lemon slices, warm water, and smooth stones to massage your feet will let you revel in your sense of touch.
- Nothing beats a massage for de-stressing. While professional bodywork feels amazing, it can also be expensive. You can self-massage many areas of your body, or ask your partner to gently work on your trouble spots. Massage oils are available at bath stores, pharmacies, and even some supermarkets.
- When getting a massage from someone else—whether your significant other or a pro—you'll be able to relax more if you do not wear your hearing aids or speech processor. Communicate your treatment preferences before getting started and arrange a hand sign or other signal to let the masseuse or masseur know that you need a change in pressure. Ask for a tap on the shoulder when you need to turn over.
- Wear soft, comfy clothes to help you relax. Warm slippers and snuggly robes are great for cooler weather.
- If you have trouble sleeping, try using a hot water bottle or a microwaveable "buddy" to help you nod off.
- Curl up on the couch in a fleece throw.
- Enjoy the warm feelings that come from petting your cat or dog.

- Keeping your head warm in winter can make your whole body feel cozy, but finding a chapeau that doesn't disturb your hearing aids or cochlear implant speech processor can be daunting. Look for one that sits high on your head to avoid generating feedback. Berets, cabbie hats, and newsboy caps are a few good choices for women, and adjustable baseball caps and fedoras are comfortable for guys.
- Dissolve bath salts in a tub of warm water and enjoy a good long soak—even better if by candlelight!

Taste

- Liven up your brown-bag lunches with homemade Mexican- or Asian-inspired dishes instead of the same-old sandwiches. Cookbooks and cooking magazines are available at the library, and many recipes are also available on the Internet—try the online version of your favorite food magazine as a starting point.
- Each time you go grocery shopping buy one new food that you have never tried before. Stick to seasonal items for the best prices.
- Try combining two soups that you have on hand, such as tomato and chicken with rice. Serve with a slice of cheese and a hunk of artisan bread for a simple and delicious dinner. You can also try mixing up breakfast cereals for variety—basic wheat flakes go with just about everything.
- Plan a meal using several different-textured foods to enjoy, such as a salad with soft spinach, crunchy walnuts, nubbly blue cheese, and chewy cranberries topped with a tangy vinaigrette.
- Add cinnamon to hot chocolate, oatmeal, or buttered toast for a little zip. Experiment with adding spices and herbs to foods you eat all the time.

Sight

- Think color! Buy inexpensive and unique coffee mugs at a dollar store or a neighborhood garage sale to wake up your kitchen.
- Bright place mats and dishtowels can also make your mealtimes more pleasant. During the long, gray days of winter, sunny yellow kitchen linens can offer cheer and the promise of spring.

- Always wear black or beige? Break out of the mold and don a scarlet scarf, a fuchsia fedora, or a turquoise t-shirt.
- Paint walls a soothing color, such as light blue or goldenrod.
- Hang vibrant posters on bare walls or in your cube at work.
- Get a bunch of silk flowers from a discount store and put them in a vase or an old jar for some no-maintenance prettiness inside throughout the year.
- The color of your sheets may help you sleep better. When the weather is hot, white or pastel sheets can make you feel a little less burdened by the high temperatures. If you have trouble falling asleep regardless of the weather, try using dark sheets, such as chocolate brown or navy blue; burrowing in these colors will give your eyes fewer distractions than lighter shades that reflect any nearby illumination.

Smell

- Simmer a few cinnamon sticks in a saucepan of water to perfume your home with this quintessential autumn scent.
- As long as you're not sensitive to fragrances, experiment with a new perfume or cologne. Many cosmetic counters offer free samples.
- Use aromatherapy candles or incense to create a calming home environment, but remember to never leave anything that you have burning unattended!
- Grind up citrus peels in the garbage disposal for a natural deodorizing effect.
- Make a list of your favorite scents and find ways to incorporate them into your life—if you love pine, for instance, go for a walk in a park. Crazy about lemon? Grate a little lemon peel onto broiled chicken for a treat at dinner.

"The Chocoholic's Imperative"

Many years ago, before I was able to afford my first hearing aids and my work options were limited, I supported myself by working as a chocolate truffle maker. What might seem like a glamorous job to the outside world was hard, back-straining manual labor on what were often thirteen- and fourteen-hour days, especially right before the December holidays and Valentine's Day.

When I would come home after chopping hundreds of pounds of chocolate and whisking gallon after gallon of Willy Wonka-inspired yumminess, eating chocolate was the last thing that I wanted to do. But I am a stereotypical female, and when stress hits I turn to chocolate. It never fails to soothe every single one of my senses.

Chocolate products—especially dark chocolate and unprocessed cocoa—are also thought to be beneficial to the cardiovascular system because they contain flavonoids, substances that have anti-oxidant properties that protect against cellular damage. Because chocolate is high in fat and calories, portion control is important, but for most people it is fine to indulge in this form of decadence as an occasional treat.[6]

While I can find a lot of gourmet chocolate out there, and some pretty "out there" flavors, too, the purist in me has always favored the simple classics. Here is a foolproof recipe for sinfully delicious chocolate truffles that you can make with grocery store ingredients and equipment that you probably already have in your kitchen.

Double Chocolate Truffles

Yield: About 50

Preparation overview: Fifteen minutes of active cooking time, then overnight refrigeration and then thirty minutes to finish the recipe.

1 package (12 ounces) semisweet chocolate chips

1 package (about 11½ ounces) milk chocolate chips

2 cups (1 pint) fresh heavy cream

1 cup (2 sticks) unsalted butter, cut into pats

1 tablespoon pure vanilla extract, or to taste

2 cups unsweetened cocoa powder or sweetened ground chocolate

Optional flavorings and add-ins (see notes)

1. Empty the chocolate chips into a large mixing bowl and set aside.

2. Pour the cream into a 2- or 3-quart heavy saucepan. Add the butter to the cream and place the saucepan over medium-high heat.

3. Bring the cream and butter to a boil, whisking frequently. Watch the mixture so that it does not boil over.

4. When the cream and butter have reached the boiling point, carefully pour the mixture over the chocolate in the bowl. Cover the bowl with a cookie sheet for about five minutes, to allow the chocolate to melt.

5. Using the whisk, stir the mixture—called ganache—until the cream is completely incorporated into the chocolate and the ganache is perfectly smooth. Start slowly so that you don't splash the cream all over the counter. As the cream and butter meld together, you can whisk more vigorously. The ganache will contain a few air bubbles.

6. Scrape the sides and bottom of the bowl with a rubber scraper or a "spoonula" to make sure that all of the chocolate is melted. Then whisk in the vanilla extract. Taste the ganache and add more vanilla if desired.

7. Seal the bowl with foil and refrigerate overnight, or until firm.

8. The next day, cover your counter with waxed paper to make cleanup easy. Empty the cocoa powder or sweet ground chocolate into a pie plate or other shallow dish. Cover a cookie sheet with parchment paper or waxed paper.

9. Using a melon baller or other small kitchen scoop, portion slightly rounded balls of the ganache from the bowl. Roll each one into a smooth ball using your hands, and then roll the smooth balls in the cocoa powder or sweet ground chocolate until completely coated. You can wear latex or vinyl gloves to make the rolling less messy. Place the truffles onto the cookie sheet so that they are not touching.

10. To serve, arrange the truffles on a pretty plate, or place each truffle in a paper candy cup and wrap several in a cellophane bag to give as a gift.

11. Refrigerate until ready to serve or give. If you have competing nonchocolate flavors such as onions or garlic in the

refrigerator, transfer the truffles to an airtight container. The truffles will keep fresh in the refrigerator for one week. Truffles can also be frozen for up to two months; thaw covered in the refrigerator overnight.

Notes

- Use the best quality ingredients for best results—real chocolate, fresh cream (no canned milk or half-and-half; the recipe won't work with these dairy products), and sweet (unsalted) butter.
- You can vary this recipe to suit just about any taste. If you prefer all dark chocolate, for instance, replace the milk chocolate chips with a second 12-ounce bag of semisweet chips or use two bags of bittersweet chips.
- For a more "grown-up" version, add 3 tablespoons (one 50 ml miniature bottle available at many liquor stores) of your favorite liqueur or flavored brandy along with the vanilla extract. The following flavors are especially good:

  crème de menthe or peppermint schnapps
  coffee-flavored liqueur, such as Kahlúa
  amaretto
  blackberry or raspberry brandy

- If you like add-ins, stir them into the ganache *after the ganache has chilled for two hours* to prevent the add-ins from sinking to the bottom of the bowl. Use 1½ cups total of any of the following:

  nuts (walnuts, almonds, hazelnuts, and pecans are excellent)
  shredded or flaked coconut
  mini chocolate chips
  raisins

- This variation got me a marriage proposal several years ago, although not from the man I eventually married. Stir 3 tablespoons of Grand Marnier or other orange-flavored liqueur into the ganache along with the vanilla extract. Add one tablespoon each of finely grated orange zest and finely grated, peeled fresh ginger (peel the ginger with a potato peeler).

Grating is quick if you use a microplane. Whisk thoroughly before chilling. The fragrance alone of this ganache will send you to the moon.

- If you want to dip the truffles into melted chocolate, omit the cocoa powder or sweet ground chocolate. Dipping chocolate needs to be "tempered," which is a process of carefully melting and cooling the chocolate before using it for dipping, so that the chocolate sets properly when it hardens. Tempering can be tricky and time-consuming, but if you want to try it, the Ghirardelli Chocolate Company has clear directions on its Web site; see appendix B for the link.

- A final note about cleanup—if there are any scrapings of chocolate left in the bowl after you finish making your truffles (not likely, but just in case), throw that chocolate into the garbage, not down the drain. Putting chocolate into a drain is like pouring sand down there, and you may wind up with a nasty sink clog. After doing the dishes, run hot water into the drain for a few seconds, to make sure that the pipes are clear.

5

To Your Health

A HIGHER PERCENTAGE of working-age people with hearing loss have chronic health conditions relative to working-age people without hearing loss. These debilitating conditions are costly on both the individual and societal levels. General practitioners and family physicians need to better address the prevention, diagnosis, and treatment of these health issues, and people with hearing loss need to be assertive in requesting appropriate care.

This chapter provides an overview of the health status of the working-age population that shows disparities in how people with and without hearing loss view their health. Differences in the prevalence of serious chronic health conditions among working-age people by hearing ability are presented, along with the costs of these conditions. A discussion of health insurance coverage by hearing category highlights how payment sources differ between people with and without hearing loss. Tips to improve communication at the doctor's office are included, followed by a lighthearted account of the author's recent experiences in primary care settings.

The Health Status of the Working-Age Population

An old saying holds that people are as healthy as they think they are, and a growing body of research lends scientific credence to that claim. Self-reported health status is a predictor of overall health, some health behaviors, and mortality risk; lower perceived health status is associated with a higher risk of dying and a higher use of medical services.[1] People with hearing loss report lower health statuses compared to people with better hearing, and they go to the

doctor more often. People with trouble hearing also have, not sur-
prisingly, trouble communicating with their health care providers.[2]
This barrier to information may contribute to health issues.

Figure 15 shows clear differences in self-reported health between
working-age people with excellent or good hearing and people
with any trouble hearing. Almost twice the percentage of people
without hearing trouble report being in excellent health (34 percent) compared to people with any hearing trouble (18 percent).
Two out of three people with better hearing—67 percent—report
being in excellent or very good health, compared to slightly fewer
than half—47 percent—of people with trouble hearing. At the other
end of the scale, 9 percent of people with excellent or good hearing

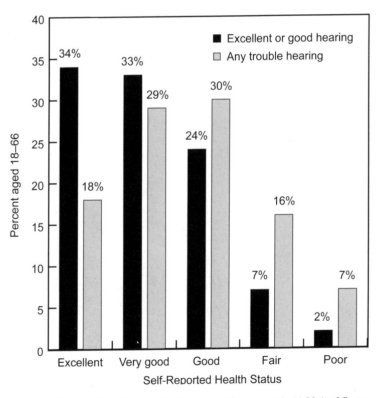

Figure 15. Reported health status by hearing ability, ages 18–66, United States,
2008. *Refused to answer, not ascertained, and don't know responses excluded.*

consider themselves to be in fair or poor health, versus 23 percent of people with hearing loss. Is hearing loss alone responsible for these disparities? Probably not. Many chronic conditions are more prevalent in the nonelderly hearing impaired population, and these health issues in combination with a hearing loss can have a compounded negative impact on overall health.

Comorbid Conditions and Hearing Loss

Diabetes is a growing health concern in the United States, regardless of hearing ability. People with diabetes are roughly twice as likely to die early compared to people of the same age without the disease, and diabetes can shorten longevity by 10 to 15 years. Medical expenses incurred by people with diabetes are more than twice as high as the health expenses of people without diabetes.[3]

Figure 16 shows that more than twice the percentage of working-age people with trouble hearing (13 percent of people with a little trouble hearing and 16 percent of people with moderate or a lot of trouble hearing) have ever been told that they have diabetes compared to people with excellent or good hearing who have been diagnosed with the disease (6 percent).

As noted in the introduction, research suggests that diabetes can trigger hearing loss by damaging nerves or blood vessels. While future research should shed more light on these processes, it appears that preventing diabetes can have a protective effect on hearing loss. People with any trouble hearing must be diligent about monitoring their health for diabetes symptoms and be sure to discuss any concerns about either condition with their health care providers.

People with hearing loss also need to be vigilant about preventing (or promptly treating symptoms of) several other health conditions. According to the Medical Expenditure Panel Survey, asthma, mental disorders (depression, anxiety, and related conditions), and hypertension are some of the most common chronic health conditions in the overall working-age population.[4] Figure 17 shows that people ages 18–66 with hearing loss have higher rates of each of these conditions relative to people without hearing trouble.

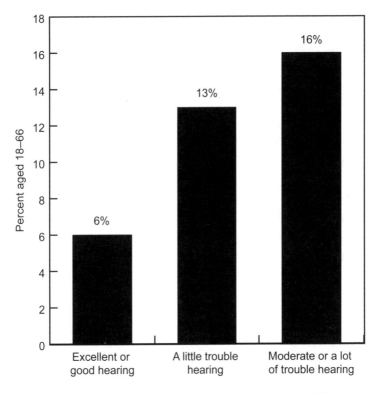

Figure 16. Percentage of the working-age population ever told by a health professional that they have diabetes, by hearing ability, United States, 2008. *Refused to answer, not ascertained, don't know, and borderline diabetes responses excluded.*

Asthma is seen in 12 percent of the working-age population with excellent or good hearing, 16 percent of people with a little trouble hearing, and 17 percent of people with moderate or a lot of trouble hearing.

Depression is more prevalent than asthma and hypertension in all working-age people. More than one in four of people ages 18–66 with better hearing—26 percent—has ever had depression, almost half—47 percent—of people in this age group with a little trouble hearing have ever had this condition, and one in two—exactly 50 percent—of people in the working ages with moderate or a lot of trouble hearing has ever had the disease.

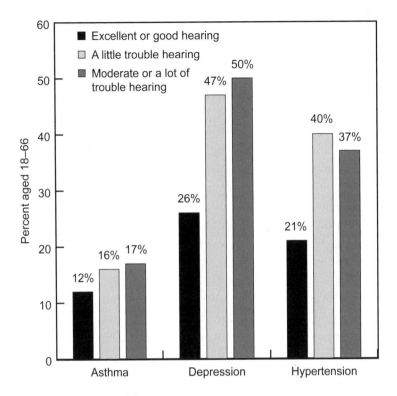

Figure 17. Percentage of people ages 18–66 who have ever had asthma, depression, or hypertension, by hearing ability, United States, 2008. *Refused to answer, not ascertained, and don't know responses excluded.*

Hypertension is also far from rare in working-age adults. Just over one in five of those people with better hearing—21 percent— have had high blood pressure, while 40 percent of people with a little trouble hearing and 37 percent of people with moderate or a lot of trouble hearing have had this condition. A higher percentage of people with a little trouble hearing have ever had hypertension relative to people with more severe hearing losses.

The 2008 National Health Interview Survey (NHIS) data set included a special module of questions on balance and dizziness, and analyses show striking differences in the rate of falling among the nonelderly population by hearing ability. Falling is generally regarded as an older-adult health issue, and very little research has been done on falls among younger population segments. This new finding hopefully will encourage researchers to look carefully at falls in the nonelderly in order to learn what causes them and to develop ways to prevent these injuries.

As shown in figure 18, 14 percent of people ages 18–49 with excellent or good hearing fell at least once in the five years before the survey, while 28 percent of the under-50 age group with a little trouble hearing experienced a fall in the same period. Thirty percent of people under 50 with moderate or a lot of trouble hearing fell during this timeframe.

The older working-age group of 50- to 66-year-olds showed the same pattern of a higher rate of falls as hearing worsened. Sixteen percent of people in this age group with better hearing fell over the previous five-year period, while 23 percent with a little trouble hearing and 30 percent with moderate or a lot of trouble hearing had fallen within five years.

Among people with a little trouble hearing, a higher proportion of younger working-age adults fell compared to older working-age adults. This intriguing finding may be due in part to more activity among younger people and consequently more exposure to the risk of falling.

Can Hearing Aids Help Reduce Depression and Falls?

Among the working-age population with hearing loss, 39 percent of those who wear a hearing aid have experienced depression, and 48 percent of those who *do not* wear a hearing aid have dealt with depression. In absolute terms, 10.2 million people ages 18–66 with hearing loss and who do not use a hearing aid have had, or currently have, this disease.[5]

Hearing aid use is also associated with a lower rate of falls among working-age people; 25 percent of the nonelderly population with any trouble hearing who wear a hearing aid have fallen at least once in the past five years while 27 percent of those with any trouble hearing who do not wear a hearing aid

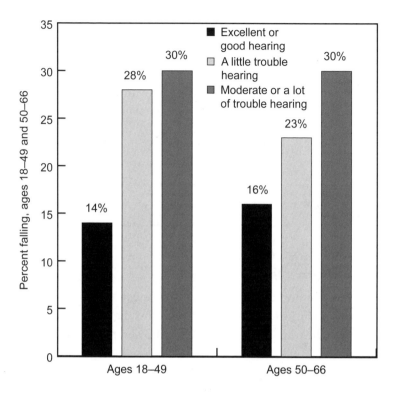

Figure 18. Percentage of people ages 18–49 and 50–66 falling unexpectedly to the floor or ground from a standing, walking, or bending position at least once in the past five years, by hearing ability, United States, 2008. *Refused to answer, not ascertained, and don't know responses excluded.*

have fallen during the same period. In absolute terms, 5.9 million working-age people with hearing loss fell, and out of this group, 5.5 million do not wear a hearing aid.[6] It is possible that falls would decrease substantially among the hard of hearing if more people in this population segment wore hearing aids.

Treating the effects of depression and falls is expensive. Average annual costs of care for mental disorders in a working-age adult were $1,517 in 2007—the most recent year for which expense data are available[7]—and the average cost of a fall among the elderly in

1999 was more than $7,000 (reliable cost data for falls in younger adults is not available).[8]

A causal relationship between hearing loss and depression, or hearing loss and falls, cannot be assumed based on these findings because the NHIS data show age ranges for hearing loss onset instead of exact ages, and determining which condition came first with precision is not possible. Also, many factors besides hearing aid use—including lifestyle behaviors, physical trauma, and medications—can explain the difference in the prevalence of depression and falling. Nonetheless, the data support the plausibility that using appropriate hearing aids will render at least some people less likely to become depressed or to fall.

Hearing Aids Have Potential for Health Care System Savings

Let's run the numbers. If hearing aid use could have prevented depression in just 10 percent of the working-age people with untreated hearing loss in the 2008 NHIS sample, at an average cost of $1,676 per hearing aid and with an average hearing aid lifespan of five years, the prorated annual cost per aid would be $335, or $1,182 less per year than the average cost of treating depression. The potential savings to the health system would be $1.2 *billion per year*—a very decent return on a hearing aid investment!

Similarly, health insurers and providers would do well to look at the possible cause-and-effect benefits of hearing health care on falls in the nonelderly. As an example, let's assume that a loss of balance causes 10 percent of falls. While limited research exists on the effects of binaural hearing aids (one in each ear) on balance, it is plausible that a person with hearing loss in both ears can have better balance if she or he uses binaural hearing aids. In this situation, using the above figures, the cost for the pair of aids would be $3,648 less than the average cost of a fall. If 10 percent of the falls among the nonelderly identified in the NHIS had been prevented with hearing aid use, the health care savings would have totaled more than $2 billion.

Could the provision of hearing health care prevent higher prevalence rates of other health conditions? Maybe. The NHIS data compellingly show that people who wear hearing aids have lower rates of depression and falls compared to people with hearing loss who do not wear hearing aids. Given the potential for better health and lower health system costs, if more extensive hearing health care does lead to fewer cases of expensive associated conditions—and perhaps a reduction in stress, which is also associated with many health issues (refer to chapter 4)—it makes sense for clinical researchers and health insurance companies to look carefully at the likely cost savings. A hearing aid costing less than $1,700 may save additional hundreds of millions of dollars in health system expenditures per year and improve the quality of life of each wearer.

Understanding the causal pathways is also important for optimizing disease prevention and treatment. As shown previously, diabetes appears to cause hearing loss in some people, but research has not yet looked at whether or not wearing hearing aids can help control diabetes. While this notion may sound far-fetched, stress can raise blood glucose levels,[9] and given the association between stress and hearing loss, it may be that untreated hearing loss is a stepping-stone to type 2 (adult-onset) diabetes.

It would also be worth investigating the benefits of cochlear implants with respect to preventing or ameliorating other health conditions. The NHIS contained very few working-age cochlear implant users, so these analyses are not possible using this data set. Other research has shown quality of life improvements in cochlear implantees,[10] though, and looking at specific health conditions among this population group could be informative for health providers.

Health Insurance by Hearing Category

In table 4 the 2008 NHIS data show that four out of five working-age adults (80 percent) with excellent or good hearing have at least one kind of health coverage, with two out of three (67 percent) having private insurance only. Medicare—for which nonelderly adults with disabilities can be eligible—is the only coverage for just 2 percent of working-age adults with better hearing. The military provides 2 percent of working-age adults with excellent or good hearing their health coverage, and another 2 percent of this segment has dual coverage (Medicare and Medicaid, or Medicare and private insurance). Medicaid—public insurance funded by the federal government and the states for lower income individuals and families—is the sole source of health insurance for 6 percent of all working-age adults, regardless of hearing ability.

Among people ages 18–66 with any trouble hearing, 16 percent lack any health insurance. More than six out of ten (62 percent) have private insurance only, with 4 percent using Medicare, and 8 percent having dual coverage. Military coverage is used by 3 percent of working-age adults with trouble hearing. The Patient

Table 4. Health insurance coverage by hearing category, ages 18–66, United States, 2008

	Excellent or Good Hearing	Any Trouble Hearing
Private only	67%	62%
Military only	2%	3%
Medicare only	2%	4%
Medicaid only	6%	6%
Dual Medicare/ Medicaid or Medicare/Private	2%	8%
No coverage	20%	16%

Military includes TRICARE, VA coverage, CHAMP-VA, and other military health care coverage. Other government programs, including Indian Health Service, are excluded because of too few responses to be statistically valid. "No coverage" means none of these types and excludes other government programs because of too few responses to be statistically valid. Refused to answer, not ascertained, and don't know responses excluded. Percentages do not add up to 100 due to rounding.

Protection and Affordable Care Act signed into law in 2010 does not mandate hearing health care, and in its current form will have no direct impact on hearing health care. With the provisions in the act to offer health coverage to people who have been denied insurance due to preexisting conditions, however, it is possible that people with hearing loss may be able to get a health plan under the law that they could not obtain earlier (health plans can consider hearing loss as a preexisting condition, even if they do not offer benefits for hearing aids). At this time, though, obtaining such a plan will not help cover hearing expenses.

Although most working-age people with hearing loss have health insurance, they still have higher out of pocket expenses than do people with excellent or good hearing. The 2008 NHIS data show that in the twelve months before the survey, 12 percent of working-age adults with excellent or good hearing, 16 percent of those with a little trouble hearing, and 17 percent of people with moderate or a lot of trouble hearing had family out-of-pocket health costs of at least $3,000.[11]

These costs exclude over-the-counter health products, insurance premiums, and reimbursed costs. Other family members' health expenses could be responsible for some or all of the difference between out-of-pocket costs reported by survey respondents with hearing loss compared to those without hearing loss, and other health conditions coexisting with a hearing loss can factor into the higher costs paid by the hard of hearing. Also, insurance benefits provided to people with excellent or good hearing may be more comprehensive on average than the benefits available to policyholders with hearing loss. As discussed in chapter 3, few health insurance plans offer coverage for hearing aids, and those that do usually pay for a just small percentage of the cost of hearing health care devices.

Tips for Better Health Care at Your Provider

Going to the doctor can be nerve-racking even without a hearing loss, but having a communications obstacle can add to the strain. Many straightforward ways can be used to smooth the process and to make your health care visits more productive and informative. With just a bit of planning and proactivity, you can help to ensure that you get the best care. The following ideas can help your appointments go well.

- Ask your health care providers for e-mailed appointment reminders instead of phone calls.
- Have each of your health care providers, including your dentist, note on the cover of your chart (or in the first field of your electronic medical record) that you are hard of hearing. Include communications requirements, such as the need for visual cues when you are called from the waiting room, the importance of facing you while talking so that you can speechread, and your inability to hear a provider when you remove your hearing aids or speech processor to have your ears examined.
- Remember the importance of preventive care, especially in light of the other health conditions that are more common in people with hearing loss. Keep up with your annual physicals and age-appropriate exams.
- Don't put off doctor visits for necessary care because you don't want to get weighed. You have the right as a patient to refuse to get on the scale.
- Make sure that your dentist or hygienist writes down instructions, or that you establish nonverbal cues for tasks (such as pantomiming when it is time to rinse). Dental light shining in your eyes can impede your ability to speechread.
- Make sure to get instructions for a mammogram or other X-ray before the technician or radiologist walks behind the safety partition. If you have a cochlear implant, magnetic resonance imaging (MRI) studies must be done under special conditions that will need to be arranged between the MRI center and your implant manufacturer to avoid damaging the implant. Never expose yourself to uncontrolled magnetic fields because they can damage your implant.
- Do as much as possible online instead of by phone—refilling prescriptions, requesting appointments, and communicating

with your health care providers online are becoming more widely available options. These steps help to reduce the demand on your ears.

- If you rely on speechreading and are having surgery, make sure to ask your doctor any questions before she puts on her surgical mask. Don't be shy about reminding nurses and other medical team members that you need to see their faces in order to "hear" what they are saying. Some surgery centers will let you wear your hearing aids or cochlear implant processors into the operating room, but if they won't, arrange with a nurse or a family member to give you your devices as soon as you get to the post-op recovery area.

Doc, It Hurts Right Hear

I had my annual physical the other day, and the good news is that it looks like I'll be around to annoy everyone for several more decades. Despite this happy (well, to me, anyway) report, I left my doctor's office with the furrowed brow I have whenever I am both flummoxed and frustrated. "Health care provider" can be an oxymoron to someone with hearing loss. My medical group is well equipped with all kinds of cool diagnostic technology that seems to do everything except self-destruct. In the waiting room are serenity-inducing paintings of happy golden retrievers, who are almost, but not quite, as cute as my hearing dog, Bogie. Nouveau amenities such as ergonomic chairs and gourmet coffee add to the nurturing ambience.

My doctor and nurse practitioner are knowledgeable and compassionate souls—really *human* human beings—but even they have been morphing into mostly digital communicators, exchanging information with each other electronically more than in person. As far as I can tell, the only 20th-century artifacts at the health center are the pictures of Tom Selleck and Robert Redford in the mammography screening room, and there is some justification for keeping those relics around. While I am campaigning for Bono and Matthew McConaughey ("Who?" the radiology technician asked, right before the mammography machine squished me as Tom and Bob watched the whole thing with their winning smiles), most of the patients are still (a little) older than I am, so I'll just have to fantasize for a few more years while the demographics shift.

But when it comes to managing the care of people with hearing disabilities, the facility is mired in the Dark Ages. In fairness, the problems are not exclusive to this one group. Every practice to which I have been assigned over the years—and there have been several, as primary care doctors have shifted and shuffled in and out of my medical plans nonstop—has been ill-equipped to communicate with me. Over the years, I have reminded myself that the *m* in HMO stands for "maintenance," not "make it better."

And let me tell you, health care providers are high-maintenance. When I checked in for my physical, I reminded the receptionist as I do every time I come in, "I am hearing impaired, and I would appreciate it if, when the nurse is ready for me, he or she could either hold up a piece of paper with my name on it instead of calling me, or actually come get me in the waiting room, because I won't hear my name being called."

"We can't do that," she responded automatically.

"Why?" I asked. "This is a medical office—how do you communicate with people who are hard of hearing?"

"I don't know. I just check people in, ma'am. The nurse will call you when he is ready for you." She handed me my copayment receipt and dismissed me with a wave of her hand. Pffthhht. I knew I wasn't going to win that battle, so I walked away and stationed myself in a comfy, good-for-my-spine chair in the waiting room with a clear line of sight to the door from where the nurse would call me. Bogie plopped down at my feet.

I watched the door and glanced occasionally at the "health for your happy life" TV monitor; if I buried myself in reading the waiting room pamphlets on hypertension and long-term care, I would miss my call for sure. There was no captioning on the TV screen—I have asked staff members about that too, and have gotten only flabbergasted stares in return—but it was easy to see that the topic du jour was shopping for nutritious foods. People who dress a whole lot nicer than I do for grocery shopping were smiling while browsing through the produce section—who knew that parsnips could cause such merriment?—and frowning while looking in the cured meats department. There were even a couple of kids who chose apples over ice cream without being threatened by their parents. I suspect that they were either really gullible or really intimidated by the show's director.

Bogie and I were watching the third run-through of the completely unrealistic food shopping video when my doctor's nurse came to the doorway. I had made the mistake of concentrating on the program and was watching a segment on whole-grain bread with rapt attention instead of focusing on the door. A robust, athletic shopper in the video was loading up on piles of brown seeds in the bulk foods section, while a pasty and somber customer put three loaves of presumably lethal white bread in his basket.

I didn't hear my name until the nurse hollered, "Okay, Sara! Third time—last call!" Wow, that got everyone's attention, especially mine. Maybe the compression in my hearing aids could be adjusted so that shouting nurses wouldn't make me jump.

I strained to smile as I said, "I didn't hear you at first, because I am hearing impaired, remember? That is why I wear hearing aids. That is why I have a hearing dog. I tell you that every time I come in. Why doesn't someone just put that in my record?"

"It's not our policy," he answered, before turning away to lead me to the examination room. He was chattering while he was walking in front of me; I could see his shoulders and head moving as he spoke, but I had no idea what he was saying. Since he was going to take my blood pressure in a couple of minutes, I didn't want to get any more ticked off than I already was and point out yet another policy mosquito that kept flying in my face. The nurse looked at me only when we stopped at the scale to get my weight.

Ooo. I hate this part. Before I got on the scale, I took off my shoes, my jacket, one sweater, Bogie's treat pouch that I wear strapped on my waist, and my watch—hey, I'm officially in middle age now, and I need every BMI break I can get—and I was debating with myself about taking out my hearing aids, but I got a dirty look from the nurse. Patience did not appear to be one of his virtues.

"Just get on the scale," he yipped. "The hearing aids don't matter," he added, from which I inferred more than one meaning that really made my day. I shut up after that; it took a supreme effort on my part, but I knew that complaining further at this level wasn't going to do any good.

(I am deliberately omitting the rest of the weigh-in episode. Onward.)

When I saw my doctor a few minutes later, I brought up the communications problems as I had so many times before, and he apologized again as he had so many times before. He told me that he would bring the issues up one more time at the next staff meeting. I offered to write a list of practices that they could implement, such as visual notification and sensitivity training for communicating with people with hearing disabilities, but he said that they had internal procedures that they had to follow instead.

"So that means," I summed up, "that I can expect bubkes to change?"

"I don't know," he said. At least he was honest. "I know that these are real problems, but they are also not priorities here. We have to pick and choose."

"Effective communication isn't a condition," I pointed out. "And I know I'm a little wacky—okay, maybe a lot wacky—but I don't think that it's nuts to expect people here to know how to communicate with patients with hearing losses. I understand what you are saying, but it doesn't make a whole lot of sense. It is hard for me to believe that I am the only patient here who has been on the receiving end of these issues. If I can help at all, just let me know."

My doctor got that look of exaggerated patience on his face that I had seen so many, many times before. "Look on the bright side, Sara" he said. "You're so healthy it's disgusting. I love your lipid profile." He held up the lab report and smiled with admiration in his eyes, and then turned away yet again to scribble in my chart.

"Well, good," I said wryly. "I can brag about my triglycerides the next time my husband and I have a date night. And it's nice to know that I should live long enough to rattle cages around here and get some changes made." My doctor was busy writing and didn't respond. "Did you hear me?" I asked.

"Huh?" He finally looked up. "Sorry, what did you say? You really have a date?"

"Never mind," I answered, using the stock response that people give me all of the time when they don't want to repeat themselves. I could feel my blood pressure shooting up, and I thought of Bogie frolicking after squirrels to calm myself down again. And I counted to ten, which may not have been a long enough pause, but my doctor chimed in again.

"Sounds good," he said. Oh, the irony. "Take care of yourself," he added. As Bogie and I walked out, I thought about my health care utopia. This will be a world where doctors and nurses face me so that I can see what they are saying, the educational videos in the waiting room are captioned, the surgical masks that my dentist wears are transparent so that I can speech read during a root canal, hearing aids and audiograms are covered by insurance, and—why not?—there are virtual dudes on demand in the mammography room. And the squishing won't hurt a bit.

6

When Silence Isn't Golden: The Hearing Health Care Backstory

AUDIOLOGISTS AND HEARING aid dispensers have difficult jobs. They make their livings selling expensive, ugly, fragile, cantankerous, easily broken, sometimes uncomfortable products that are a hassle to use, costly to maintain, and a long way from a cure for hearing loss. They have to market to a reluctant group, many members of which would rather eat glass than buy and use hearing aids.

Take me for an example. I have the epitome of a love/hate relationship with my hearing aid and cochlear implant. Over the past 20 years, I have bought five different pairs of hearing aids, with technologies ranging from entry-level in-the-ear analog aids (in that wonderful "old lady beige" color) to I-think-there's-a-self-destruct-button-on-these-digital-behind-the-ear-gold-sparkle-that-can-talk-to-each-other aids. Two years ago, I had cochlear implant surgery on one ear, and the titanium-encased bionics now permanently attached to my skull continue to amaze me throughout the day. The Bionic Woman from the 1970s television series has nothing on me now! I love that scientific breakthroughs have enabled me to continue living in the hearing world. I hate that my electronic ears are so expensive and cumbersome.

I am not alone. Other working-age people feel the same way. The cost of the devices presents a huge barrier to hearing aid use. Despite the benefits (refer to chapter 5), only about 7 percent of the working-age, hard of hearing population in the United States wear hearing aids.[1] Among the working-age population who have or have had a hearing aid but are not using one now, or who have had a hearing aid recommended, almost one third of men (32 percent) and close to half of women (49 percent) do not use a hearing aid because the devices cost too much.[2]

In addition to the price of hearing aids, the purchase process is fraught with inefficiencies, fragmentation, and disconnects that make buying, programming, and repairing a hearing aid a time-consuming and pricey nightmare for the consumer. As was noted in a Hearing Industries Association white paper, "The hearing health care delivery system in the United States has many interrelated issues that make access confusing, difficult and expensive."[3]

Make no mistake: Selling hearing aids is a for-profit enterprise, just like all other facets of the health care system in the United States. The precedent of a consumer paying for hearing aids entirely out of pocket has existed since health insurance began in this country in the 1920s, and the custom has persisted as widespread third-party insurance coverage excludes hearing aids today. While some health insurance plans and government programs now offer benefits for hearing health care as described in chapter 3, the sums for reimbursement are typically well below the retail cost of the devices.

When my doctor told me that I needed hearing aids all those years ago, I was stunned to find out that this medical equipment was not covered by my insurance. It turned out that this explicit exclusion in the fine print of most policies was the rule, not the exception, in U.S. health plans. I started asking people in the health care industry why. I called insurance agents; I wrote health insurance company chief executive officers; I talked to benefits representatives at company open enrollment fairs; and, in recent years, I e-mailed analysts at health insurance companies the question, "Why doesn't your policy cover hearing aids?"

Responses have fallen into two categories. Letters and e-mails without exception have generated a permanent silence. No response. Nothing. Zippo. Zilch. In person I have always gotten a blank stare, followed by words like, "I don't know. I don't think that they're medically necessary."

It dawned on me that these people did not know the answer. Several years ago, I started researching the matter, and I found a lot of intriguing policies and practices in my review of hundreds of reports, papers, and government documents. This chapter presents these findings, from the perspective of the consumer, not from those of the provider or the hearing aid manufacturer.

First, a short history of hearing health care provides chronological context for understanding the problems in the industry today. Next, a discussion of the providers in hearing health care illustrates the competing interests of audiologists and doctors and how these interests can affect patient care because of competition, greed, and process inefficiencies. The chapter concludes with an anecdote showing that however nutty life can be with hearing aids, it can still put a smile on your face.

A (Very Brief) History of Hearing Health Care

Health insurance as we know it had its beginnings in the United States in 1929 when Baylor University Hospital offered schoolteachers up to three weeks of hospital care each year for $6 per month (about $76.00 in 2009 dollars).[4] As the Depression started, teachers were assured protection from catastrophic financial loss because of illness. This health care model grew to other states in the 1930s, developing into what we still know of as Blue Cross and Blue Shield and eventually becoming regulated by many individual states.

Reimbursement-based health insurance followed in the late 1930s, and employer-sponsored plans began during World War II. When fringe benefits were exempted from wage freezes in 1942, insurance benefits became a way to attract workers to firms during wartime. By the end of the war, Blue Cross had 26 million members—over one-sixth of the U.S. population at the time—and employer-sponsored health insurance continued to grow in popularity during peacetime. Health insurance premiums paid by employers have been officially tax-free since 1954.[5]

During the twenty-five years that the health insurance industry was in its infancy, childhood, and adolescence, hearing aids were also in the early stage of development. The few manufacturers that were making the devices were often firms that also produced radios and other electric products far removed from the health care realm. In other words, hearing aids were not considered to be mainstream health care devices during this period, and so they were not covered benefits in health insurance plans. In 1935 and 1936, surveys conducted by the U.S. Public Health Service documented the extent of hearing loss in this country, and this information led to the development of improved hearing aids and, in 1941, a vocational rehabilitation manual published by the U.S. Office of Education with information specific to the employment of people who were Deaf or hard of hearing.[6]

Hearing Aids in the Military

During World War II, hearing loss existing in recruits and acquired by soldiers during active duty catalyzed the development of a large-scale hearing health care system in the military, called the Military Aural Rehabilitation Programs. The first facility was established at Walter Reed Hospital in 1943 with additional centers opening in different regions in the United States in the following years.

Some 14,000 men were treated at these facilities. They received hearing aids, speech reading instruction, vocational support, and ancillary medical care under the direction of an otologist who supervised a team of specialists including acoustic technicians, psychologists, educational counselors, and Red Cross workers who helped boost the morale of deafened troops.[7]

The benefits of treating hearing loss became clear. Veterans were able to be retrained into new, productive careers; their psychological makeup improved; and their overall quality of life was better when their hearing losses were managed and when they had the support of a health care team comprised of audiologists, speech pathologists, and physicians specializing in the treatment of the ear.

The Military Aural Rehabilitation Programs also established a system of testing hearing aids to determine the best models for its patients. The programs worked with the patient in multiple fitting sessions and offered extensive aural rehabilitation to maximize the benefits that the patient could get from the aid. The programs purchased hearing aids via contracts with manufacturers, and samples were available at the treatment centers, which gave patients as short a wait time as possible for their devices. Soldiers were also instructed in the care of their hearing aids and given enough batteries to last for the first month.[8]

Today, the Department of Veterans Affairs (VA) is the largest single customer of hearing aids in the United States, accounting for 17 percent of all sales.[9] The VA and the Army also have implemented hearing conservation programs that have collectively saved more than $874 million by decreasing hearing loss in soldiers and civilians between 1974 and 1997.[10]

Hearing Aids in the Private Sector

Beltone began manufacturing hearing aids in 1940, marketing its products in *The Saturday Evening Post, National Geographic*, and other publications with grand slogans:

Find out why the DEAF call it a miracle

World's Smallest Hearing Aid! SO SMALL it slips into a man's watch pocket

deafness [sic] Nearly Cost Me MY JOB! . . . until I discovered this New "Invisible Electronic Ear!"[11]

Until transistors were incorporated into hearing aids in 1954, devices were body-worn and much bigger than today's products. Zenith was a major manufacturer of hearing aids, marketing a $40 model in 1943 ($500 in 2009 dollars) and transistor models costing up to $125 ($1,008 in 2009 dollars) in 1954 and 1955. Hearing aids were sold through the mail and over the counter, with bricks-and-mortar dealerships becoming more common starting in 1956.[12]

The Senate Judiciary Subcommittee on Antitrust and Monopoly investigated the high prices of hearing aids in 1962, which resulted in Zenith, Beltone, and other firms releasing price and sales information as part of the investigation.[13] The first day of hearings, Eleanor Roosevelt testified before the committee, "I have a great many complaints from people who have bought hearing aids and found them not suitable to them because they went on an advertisement without having consulted a doctor or a clinic."[14] Mrs. Roosevelt's words and the rest of the investigation were the catalysts for later regulations that classified hearing aids as medical devices.

Hearings and testimony also provided details of the quackery and disingenuous business practices that flourished in the hearing aid market of the 1950s and early 1960s. Many hearing aid customers were duped into buying expensive products that did little or nothing to help their hearing losses. Congressional testimony reported that, "Unscrupulous dealers are able to profit because few hearing aid buyers know anything about the product they need," and an instruction manual for hearing aid salespeople told them "to ask prospective buyers if they have noticed a hearing loss. If the answer is 'No,' the salesman is instructed to lower his voice and continue talking."[15]

These problems were also noticed at the state level. Oregon became the first state to require the certification of hearing aid dealers and salespeople when it passed an act to this effect in 1959,[16] but despite the awareness of shady hearing aid dealers, Oregon was the only state to have this form of consumer protection until 1965 when Medicare became law.

During Congressional testimony prior to Medicare's enactment, hearing aid manufacturers lobbied vigorously against hearing aids being included in Medicare's package of benefits. Representatives from these firms disputed the rationality of, for example, economies of scale (that, as described earlier, were already used in the military), which would result from increased sales volume generated by higher demand.

The supply side argued that people who were hearing impaired were the true barriers to growth efficiencies because they typically delayed buying hearing aids for several years after they were diagnosed with a hearing loss due to vanity. Manufacturers also cited low profit margins throughout the distribution channel, attributable in large part to the lengthy amount of time that dispensers had to spend with each hearing aid purchaser.[17] (Today, the time a practitioner spends on advising patients is still cited as a justification for the high prices of hearing aids.)[18] As a result of successful lobbying, Medicare was enacted with an explicit exclusion for hearing aids that remains to this day.[19]

The bracketing out of hearing aids from mainstream medicine continued until the 1970s, when the House Subcommittee on Health and Long-Term Care of the Select Committee on Aging reported that, "The hearing aid delivery system, as presently structured, fosters a clear and continuing conflict of interest that pits the profit orientation of the businessmen who sell hearing aids against the health and economic interests of elderly consumers. . . . There is almost a total lack of oversight and scrutiny of the hearing aid industry."[20]

As a result of these and past committee hearings, the Medical Device Act of 1976 mandated the regulation of hearing aids as medical devices by the U.S. Food and Drug Administration (FDA) starting in 1977. Since then, the agency has regulated hearing aids as prosthetic medical devices that provide therapeutic benefits to hearing. Any company or person involved in the manufacture or sale of hearing aids must comply with the FDA regulations for these products in order to protect the patients who use this form of health care. The act established strict requirements for the dispensing of hearing aids, including the provision of the user instructional brochure that dispensers are still required to give with each hearing aid purchase.

The legislation mandated either the completion of a physician's examination prior to a hearing aid purchase or a waiver of the examination, but the original intent of the waiver was to accommodate people with personal values that went against medical examinations and the exceptional circumstance where a patient did not have ready access to a doctor. The waiver, therefore, was not designed to accelerate the purchase process.[21] Specifically, "the purpose of the medical evaluation by a licensed physician is to assure that all medically treatable conditions that may affect hearing are accurately identified and properly treated before a hearing aid is bought."[22]

The Role of Audiologists

Before 1979 audiologists were not allowed to dispense hearing aids because of ethical concerns,[23] and the distinction between audiologists and hearing aid dispensers was an absolute one. After the FDA assumed oversight of hearing aids as medical devices in 1977, however, a group of audiologists founded the Academy of Dispensing Audiologists "to foster and support the professional dispensing of hearing aids by qualified audiologists in rehabilitative practices."[24] With the new profit potential, audiologists understandably wanted to capitalize on their expertise. Because state-level hearing aid dispenser laws were on the books at this point, audiologists needed to become licensed hearing aid dispensers as well, which is why one practitioner, depending on a state's laws, can be both an audiologist and a hearing aid dispenser.

In addition to the regulatory distinction between dispensers and audiologists, substantial training disparities exist too. As history has shown, the hearing aid dispenser has evolved as a member of a sales force, with a less health-oriented background and approach than an audiologist. The audiologist, in comparison, has developed as part of a paramedical profession since the mid-20th century, becoming "a specialist in normal and impaired hearing and balance who provides assessment, fitting, and orientation of hearing aids and other assistive devices."[25]

Until recently, audiologists were required to have a graduate, but not necessarily a doctoral, degree for certification by the American Speech-Language-Hearing Association (ASHA; the primary certifying entity for audiologists in the United States),[26] but states are transitioning to a doctoral degree as the minimum educational requirement for an audiology license. As of January 1, 2012, ASHA will certify only doctoral degree holders.[27]

In practice, the standards for a doctorate in audiology (AuD) degree have been muddy, although they are becoming clearer. Audiologists now holding the AuD degree may have acquired this designation through distance learning that offered credit for work experience after they were already working in the field (with master's degrees); from traditional residential academic programs;[28] or by a now-defunct process called Earned Entitlement (EE), by which a practicing audiologist with a master's degree could obtain the AuD designation by offering evidence to the Audiology Foundation of America (AFA) that his or her acquired experience was equivalent to that of an earned doctorate in the field. ASHA deemed this practice unethical in 1997, and the AFA stopped granting EE-based AuD degrees in 1999.[29]

Whether this change is good for the consumer is debatable. The profession constructed the AuD degree in an effort to render audiology a doctoring profession that will facilitate its members to become "limited license practitioners," or LLPs. With this status, audiologists have a better chance at achieving their long-sought goal of what is called "direct access," which will allow patients to see audiologists directly—without having to see a physician first. Direct access will also enable audiologists to bill third-party payers (insurance companies and Medicare), and advocating for direct access is a "Highest Priority" objective of ASHA.[30] In sum—and in theory—"The public benefits from the quality of care resulting from Doctor of Audiology programs, and the Doctor of Audiology enjoys the recognition, acceptance, prestige and economic rewards associated with a doctoring profession."[31]

Audiologists and the American Academy of Otolaryngology–Head and Neck Surgery (AAO-HNS), an organization for medical doctors who specialize in ear care, among other areas of the head and neck, have been grappling with direct access for quite a while. Medical doctors do not agree with audiologists that direct access is in the best interest of the patient. The AAO-HNS posits that "hearing and balance disorders are medical issues, and require a full patient history and examination by a physician."[32] ASHA and another organization of audiologists, the American Academy of Audiology, have introduced legislation to expand their turf through direct access.[33] If direct access is implemented, a patient will not have to have an examination by a physician prior to getting hearing aids. Consider the economic ramifications: Audiologists will probably enjoy an increase in their business, and doctors may have a decrease in their billable charges because of patients going directly to audiologists.

Is direct access good for the patient with a hearing loss? As a consumer who has been treated by no fewer than twenty audiologists over the last thirty years—about a third of whom have doctoral degrees—I think that these practitioners are very good at testing hearing and fitting hearing aids. Most of them have been conscientious and responsive, but I do not think of audiologists as doctors.

While my experience is admittedly not scientific and is only anecdotal, I have not found that doctoral-level audiologists' training and skills are as well developed as those of the medical doctors whom I have seen about my hearing loss, and I do not think that AuD holders are qualified to diagnose or treat any ear disorders that I may develop. In the hundreds of hours that I have spent being treated by audiologists, the master's-level practitioners have provided care and offered knowledge at least as good as have the doctoral-level practitioners. In sum, in my experience, the extra education required for the AuD has not resulted in better care.

In addition, requiring a doctoral degree may unnecessarily restrict the supply of audiologists, an outcome that would not be in the best interest of the consumer. AuD degrees take about four years to complete, compared to two years for master's degrees. There were 856 master's degrees and only 19 clinical doctoral degrees in audiology conferred in the 1999–2000 school year,[34] but the balance shifted dramatically in the next eight years. Degree-granting institutions conferred 97 master's degrees and 1,154 doctoral degrees in audiology and hearing sciences in the 2007–2008 school year.[35]

The explosion in doctoral degrees, however, is not due entirely to newly minted audiologists entering the profession. Because of the transition to the doctoral degree standard, many existing master's-level audiologists are upgrading their academic qualifications to the doctorate.[36] There were roughly 12,800 existing audiologists in the field as of 2008,[37] and for this number to serve just the working-age, hard of hearing population, each practitioner would have to serve about 1,800 patients. Obviously, as shown in the introduction, many people never see an audiologist. However, as has also been shown, few people with hearing loss get amplification, and a limited supply of providers will not help the situation.

It is also possible that AuDs will charge more for their services than will master's-level hearing health care providers. That's great for them, but not for me, since I, as a consumer, will have to pay this premium. Since the value added of an AuD over a master's level audiologist's training has not been significant in my experience, I cannot help but question the economic soundness of a mandatory doctoral degree from the patient's vantage point.

Marketing, Marketing, Marketing

Hearing aid dispensers do everything that they can to get you to spend money in their offices. An article in one professional journal urges that the reception area needs to be a place "where the patient is exposed to literature about different types of hearing aids, assistive technology, batteries, and any other product or service that your practice offers."[38] Other marketing tactics advocated in the professional literature include promotional offers, coupons, direct mail advertising, and (interestingly) telemarketing.[39] Some other types of health care, such as optometry chains that send out coupons in the mail, also use these strategies, but from the consumer's perspective, these practices can come across as anything but "doctoring" in nature.

Other firms are developing large-scale marketing plans to mass-market hearing aids in big-box retailers and groceries. Strategies to increase market share and profits include having licensed dispensers on site only occasionally[40] (which will save an employer substantial labor costs) and lobbying the FDA to reclassify some hearing aids as over-the-counter models, because, "the potential market size of $5 Billion [sic] would justify the lobbying investment."[41] To date, the FDA has not approved over-the-counter hearing aids. Any "sound-amplifying device intended to compensate for impaired hearing"[42] is a hearing aid that requires a patient to have a medical evaluation, or to waive the examination, prior to purchasing the device. The FDA makes the distinction between hearing aids and "personal sound amplification products," or PSAPs; the latter are designed for people with normal hearing who want amplification for everyday activities.[43]

Another issue concerns payment mechanisms. Audiologists are aware that patients who have insurance can be less profitable to serve than those patients who pay completely out-of-pocket,[44] because "most third-party payers are notorious for reduced fees and late payments."[45] Cash patients are also preferable from an administrative viewpoint, because payment is immediate, and it takes a lot less paperwork to process self-paying patients compared to billing insurance and waiting for reimbursement.[46] Perhaps audiologists, if they want to be recognized as doctors, need to start behaving more like doctors by accepting the reimbursement schedules of third-party payers.

Audiologists also need to run their businesses more efficiently. As noted earlier, the labor-intensive process of fitting hearing aids has been used to justify high prices for a long time. What is striking is how few efficiency improvements have been made to the hearing aid purchasing process. Following are two examples of these wasteful practices, along with possible solutions to streamline the purchase process and make it simpler and more cost-effective for all parties.

Programming Hearing Aids and Cochlear Implant Speech Processors

An audiologist had me return five times for programming a new pair of hearing aids because the programming software was not correctly loaded onto her computer, the cables connecting the programming computer to my aids were not the right ones, and the audiologist had not been trained in the use of the programming software. It is understandable that new programming software requires a learning curve, but practitioners need to know their products or hire people who are more fluid in programming.

Audiologists could test patients' hearing and recommend hearing aids, and outsource the programming to people who are more skilled in that specialty.

Cochlear implant programming is especially complex. Half of the implant audiologists whom I have seen since my surgery have had to call the implant manufacturer after I have arrived for a programming appointment because they didn't know how to completely program my implant's processor. They blamed the manufacturer for making the software too complex, saying that it was designed for engineers instead of audiologists.

They were articulating the solution right there—have programmers program and let dispensers focus on what they do best, which, in my experience is not programming hearing aids or speech processors. Increased specialization can lead to less wasted time, less frustration, and overall improved efficiency from a business model perspective.

This issue goes beyond competence and extends into trust. How confident would you feel if you went to a dental appointment and your dentist told you that she did not know how to use the X-ray machine? It is not unrealistic to expect licensed professionals to thoroughly know their jobs, particularly if they call themselves doctors. At present, ASHA certification requires no specific competency standards for software programming used in hearing health care.[47]

Communicating with Patients

One practitioner told me recently that her practice does not offer online communications (beyond initial contact requests from the company Web site) because most people with hearing loss, according to this professional, do not use the Internet. For people in the working ages with hearing loss, the Internet is a saving grace on a daily basis, offering a way to send and receive information without having to worry about incorrectly hearing details on the phone. Hearing health dispensers need to set up secure online communications systems, including real-time chatting with customer service representatives to check on the status of an order, electronic appointment setting, and secure messaging with providers.

This issue is critical for postsurgical cochlear implantees. When I had my implant operation, the only after-hours communications option I had was the telephone, so my fiancé played "monkey in the middle" as a translator when I had a question for the doctor on call. It was frustrating for everyone, and it could have easily been prevented with online communications.

In sum, the efficiency of the hearing health care delivery system can be improved if the supply of audiologists is increased by removing the doctoral requirement, task specialization is adopted in dispensing offices, communications are transitioned to be more electronic and less telephone-based, and consumer-based quality-of-care standards are established and enforced. Greater government oversight to catalyze improvement in these areas may be necessary, especially with "the Silent Avalanche" of more hard of hearing people coming in future decades. Leaders need to take action now to repair an imbalanced delivery system that favors providers at the expense of patient care. With practical, realistic changes, hearing health care can provide well-organized service and helpful products at prices that are profitable to practitioners and affordable to consumers.

The Elton John Test

In case you haven't already figured this one out, I can drive audiologists a little nuts, and not just with my policy nitpicking. Bogie, my wonderful hearing dog, can help me cheat on hearing tests by using his "ear language" to tell me when the beep tones go off. Also, I have long since memorized the "baseball, cowboy, ice cream, hot dog, airplane" list of words, along with lots of those, "Say the word [fill in the blank with something impossible to understand]" auditory assessments. Since the ear pros picked up on my dog's completely natural and understandable—albeit unintentional but dare I say, very cool—talent, Bogie's place in the audiogram testing booth has been relegated to sitting behind me;

and since the canine cheating was discovered, I have had to keep my eyes closed during hearing tests.

The list memorization thing—also accidental, I swear—almost sent my otolaryngologist into a hissy fit when I mentioned it to him in passing. I have a fond memory of his galled reaction when I told him about the word lists that I could rattle off almost without thinking about them. He called my audiologist while I was in his office and told her pointedly that she needed to come up with new groups of words for me so that my test results would be accurate.

Ah, wonderful, more words that I could not hear, but that's beside the point. Lately, with Bogie's and my behavior during hearing evaluations now censure-free, and the results even more bummer-inducing, the routine has gotten old. After about three decades of going to hearing tests, hearing aid programming sessions, and checkups, I try to proactively find ways to make my hours in the soundproof booth a little more interesting and a little less onerous.

Enter The Elton John Test (EJT). I should say right now, to pre-clude any music industry lawyers from sending my publisher or me irate e-mails, that this test does not involve canine or human trickery or deception, nor copyright infringement of any kind, and it should probably—properly—be called The Elton John/Bernie Taupin Test (Bernie Taupin has been the lyricist for most of Sir Elton's songs), but I shortened the title in a rare attempt to be pithy. And EJ/BTT looked a little weird, like a classification in a government document. No offense to the wordsmith.

I am one of the duo's biggest fans. *Captain Fantastic and the Brown Dirt Cowboy* is my all-time favorite album, and the CD was the first one that I played after my cochlear implant activation—and even though I can't hear all of the music anymore, I still know the words of most of the earlier songs by heart, thanks to the lyrics being printed in the album notes.

The EJT is simple and effective, and it can be done at home or in an audiologist's office. After I get my hearing aids or implant processor reprogrammed, I listen to some of Sir Elton's songs and compare how the music sounds to how I remember it sounding circa 1975. I take notes—lots of notes—and then I report my findings back to my audiologist in musical terms. Or sometimes I use an Excel spreadsheet if I am in an especially anal mood when I conduct the EJT. Laugh all you want (or try to get me committed), but the EJT results help to refine my device programming better than any other method I have tried over many, many years.

How does it work? As examples, where some of Ray Cooper's or Nigel Olsson's awesome percussion is lost on me when I listen to "Bitter Fingers," I let my audiologist hear that part of the song so that the aid settings can be adjusted to compensate as much as possible. If one of Davey Johnstone's killer riffs in "(Gotta Get A) Meal Ticket" is too soft or metallic to my ears, making appropriate changes to the programming becomes a lot more straightforward. And while Dee Murray's bass usually comes through at least a little, if it sounds warbled or if I feel it vibrating on "Someone Saved My Life Tonight," having the EJT data available makes modifying the low frequencies on my equipment a simpler task for my audiologist.

I realize that it may seem a little crazy to use music to improve hearing aid fittings, but hey, it works. Audiologists can hear a lot better than I ever will, and most of them listen to music and so know the sounds and adjustments to make when I use the EJT analogies. The EJT can also be modified to work with, say, Led Zeppelin, Barbra Streisand, The Beatles, Chris Isaak, or Luther Vandross, so anyone's musical tastes can be accommodated. I haven't tried it with rap yet, but that music is on my list too. (I also haven't tried it with country, but that genre is definitely not on my list. Someone else will have to give it a try and let me know how it works.)

The EJT makes the process of hearing device programming as close to enjoyable as it probably ever can be, with the result being better-programmed electronic ears. Audiologists seem to like listening to music while they are programming hearing aids and speech processors—what a concept, huh?—and the EJT has spared my doctor another conniption.

Well, at least for now. I forewarn the good doctor: Come April Fools' Day, keep your eyes open and watch your back. An intrepid dog may be behind you.

7

Going to the Dogs: The Low-Tech Advantage in a High-Tech World

CAN A DOG'S furry ears and warm heart help your sound awareness during everyday activities? Hearing service dogs—or hearing ear dogs, signal dogs, or just hearing dogs, as they are sometimes called—are specially trained to alert their guardians to sounds including alarm clocks, doorbells and knocks, telephones, and smoke alarms. Having a hearing dog is associated with increased social integration, self-esteem, and self-sufficiency; and reduced depression, anxiety, and loneliness. A service dog can also reduce reliance on both paid and volunteer help.[1]

The first hearing dog training program in the United States started in Minnesota in 1973, when the Minnesota Humane Society approached dog trainer Agnes McGrath to train six hearing dogs with funding provided by the Minnesota Lions. Three years later, the American Humane Association established a hearing dog training center in Colorado, and McGrath obtained funding to perform a hearing dog pilot study there involving herself and fellow hearing dog pioneers Martha Foss, Sandi Sterker, and Emlynn Wood. The success of that pilot program in 1979 led to the establishment of what is now the International Hearing Dog Inc. program in the greater Denver area, and many others throughout the world.[2]

A hearing service dog alerts by running back and forth between the sound source and her or his guardian until the guardian goes to the sound. A smaller hearing dog will jump up on his human's leg to give a tactile alert when a sound goes off, while a larger dog will nudge her human with her nose or her paw. Sounds for

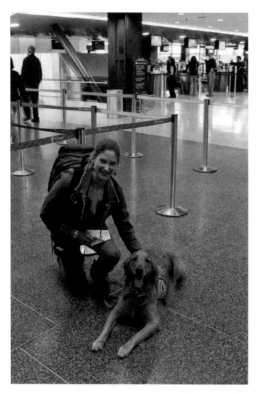

The author and her hearing dog, Bogie, ready to go through security at the Sea-Tac Airport in Seattle, Washington. Photo credit: © 2008 John S. Batinovich. All rights reserved.

which signal dogs can be trained are kitchen timers, a ringing telephone, a smoke alarm, the doorbell or a knock, a person's name, and keys dropping on the floor. While most sounds to which hearing dogs respond are in the home, the dogs also provide sound awareness outside, in work environments, on public transportation, and through that wonderful and inimitable "ear language." Train whistles, ATM beeps, and even silverware clattering on a restaurant floor are all sounds to which a hearing dog will react reflexively, giving her guardian newfound consciousness of, and confidence living in, routine surroundings.

How Hearing Dogs Differ from Guide and Other Service Dogs

While most people are familiar with guide dogs for people with visual disabilities, hearing dogs differ from guide and assistance dogs in several important ways. First, the key function of a hearing service dog is to alert his or her guardian to specific sounds, not to guide a person in the home or public places, nor to assist a human partner with physical activities such as opening a door. While all hearing dogs are well trained in basic obedience, an ongoing leadership exchange happens between a hearing dog and her guardian—the dog is in charge when a sound goes off and the dog needs to alert his or her human partner, but the human is leading the pack the rest of the time.

This balance of power is constantly shifting, and when a well-matched team communicates in synchronized harmony, the experience of seeing the beauty of partners who read each other so well is a joy for everyone involved. Each partner helps the other, and people who see them work together can appreciate the powerful benefits of a canine and human partnership.

Second, hearing dogs have very high activity levels, hair-trigger responsiveness, and curious temperaments, all essential qualities for investigating and responding to sounds. They definitely do not possess the mellow demeanors of guide or mobility assistance dogs. Energetic by nature, these dogs need the outlet of responding to signals that their job requires. Even little hearing dogs tend to be bouncy and playful, and potential guardians need to regard these traits as assets, not liabilities.

Finally, signal dogs come in all different breeds (including mixed breeds) and sizes because they are often trained by non-profit organizations that rescue from shelters dogs with the potential to become service animals. Many guide and other service dogs are, in contrast, bred specifically for their work. Several hearing dog training agencies have their hearing dog trainers visit animal shelters to assess the qualities in dogs who are available for adoption—such as sociability, reactions to sudden noises, and inquisitiveness—and who are often at risk of being euthanized because of space limitations.

Training agencies adopt canines showing promise as hearing dogs and provide shelter, health care, and training to the dogs until they are placed with their new hearing impaired guardians. Training a hearing dog takes about six months, depending on both the dog's learning curve and the program. Most training agencies have a list of sounds for which all dogs are trained to respond, and they encourage guardians to teach their canine partners to respond to additional sounds at home after formal training is complete. The methods used to train hearing dogs vary both by training agency and by the individual dog; hearing dog trainers are gifted in their abilities to bring out the best in each canine and to find the most suitable human partner for each hearing dog. Ultimately, the goal of a training program is to successfully place each hearing dog with the most appropriate guardian.

Life with a Hearing Dog

Hearing dogs perform amazing work for their human partners, but they are not for everyone with a hearing impairment. Someone who is not fond of dogs will likely find it difficult to bond with a canine partner. Signal dogs require daily practice along with all other routine care, especially the provision of a high-quality diet, exercise, playtime, grooming, and regular veterinary checkups. Applicants must have the desire and the ability to make a lifetime commitment to both the dog and to their canine/human partnership.

Even when signal dogs are properly trained and their training is maintained, they are reliable but not perfect. A guardian can expect a great deal of help with routine sound awareness on a day-to-day basis, and a rapid response if the smoke alarm goes off. But it is unlikely that a hearing dog will ever be called upon to save his guardian's life, even though he is trained to alert his human partner to a smoke alarm. A house fire isn't likely to happen whether or not someone has a hearing dog. It is important to want and appreciate a signal dog for her everyday assistance and companionship in addition to the emergency alerting skills for which she has been trained.

Hearing dogs attract constant attention in public places, which can be distracting and difficult to manage for someone uncomfortable with being repeatedly approached by people who ask questions about the dog—and the human's hearing loss. Complete strangers can be very inquisitive. Also, the high-energy personalities of hearing dogs bring immense joy to their partners' worlds, but these dogs tend to be perennial three-year-olds, with their joie de vivre manifesting as canine antics throughout their lives. They cannot be turned off, and they are not lap dogs!

Once in a while a sound out on the street such as a car alarm may cause repeated alerts that a human might rather ignore, but a hearing dog will not give up until his partner responds to his nudging. Hearing dogs, like all other dogs, live in a world based on experiences, which is not a world governed by the clock or a maximum number of tries. Hearing dogs are analogous to baseball players in this way, and persistence pays off for both. Halloween can be especially fun. Bogie, my glorious hearing dog, is enchanted by the idea that *people* get treats when the doorbell rings that one evening a year, and he is only too happy to respond to that signal a dozen times in a row on the holiday.

All Set to Get a Hearing Dog?

While it is possible to self-train a hearing dog "from scratch," the process is intensive and demanding, and it requires abilities in specialized dog training. Most people who want hearing dogs instead request an application from an agency that trains and places these magnificent service animals. Applications require a great deal of background information and verification of the applicant's hearing loss from a doctor or an audiologist.

Training programs may also ask specific questions about applicant preferences for a hearing dog's physical characteristics. Agencies will match an approved applicant with a hearing dog who meets requested criteria as closely as possible and will refrain from placing a dog with an applicant who has an incompatible wish list. A person who has a long list of preferences—for example, someone who wants only a brown, female terrier who weighs no more than twenty pounds—may be placed on a long waiting list, or never receive a hearing dog at all. Someone who is open to being matched with any dog as long as the chemistry between the dog and the human is good, however, may be matched with a canine partner within a few months after the agency approves his or her application. Waiting times vary by program but range from a few months to a few years.

In addition to considering the characteristics of each dog, training agencies carefully match applicants to canine partners based on daily routines and needs. Success with a hearing dog depends as much on the human's lifestyle as it does on the abilities of the hearing dog, and on the strength of the bond between dog and human. A person with a hearing loss who lives in an apartment, for instance, may do better with a smaller dog, while an active applicant who has a large yard can provide the exercise necessary for a larger canine partner.

As part of the application process, a representative of the training agency will inspect a potential guardian's home and interview the applicant and everyone else living with the applicant in order to learn more about daily routines, listening environments, attitudes about dogs in general, and specific expectations and goals for having a hearing dog. Training agencies will work with a new human/canine team intensively at first, showing the human how to work with her new partner at home, at work, and in public places, and making sure that the dog is doing her job. Trainers will also give instructions on feeding, grooming, and general health care. After placement, trainers will follow up with the team for the life of the dog, conducting occasional home visits and brush-up training to ensure that both members of the team are doing their jobs, and that the partnership is happy and productive. Training agencies can also require a hearing dog guardian to submit periodic written progress reports.

Most training agencies do not charge a fee for hearing dogs. Donors or community organizations often pay the costs, and legislators have recognized the worth of hearing dogs and considered providing funding for their training. In 1978, U.S. Representative Frederick W. Richmond (D-NY) and twenty-two cosponsors introduced a bill to provide funds to hearing dog training agencies; the bill was referred to the Committee on Interstate and Foreign Commerce but did not become law.[3]

While donations pay for most hearing dog training programs, often applicants pay a nominal application fee or charges for initial training classes. Once a hearing dog is placed with her guardian, the guardian assumes all costs of the dog's care. A training agency may ask a guardian to assume this financial responsibility in writing. Hearing dogs trained by service dog agencies will be spayed or neutered prior to placement.

Just as employees of a responsible training agency will be diligent in their selection of appropriate hearing dog recipients, applicants need to do their homework on the agency as well. No universal requirements or criteria exist that trainers or programs must satisfy, and training agencies are likewise unregulated. A reliable source of information for people considering a hearing dog is Assistance Dogs International (ADI), based in Santa Rosa, California. ADI's mission is the development and implementation of, and adherence to, consistent standards for service dog training and placement.

Members of ADI are nonprofit groups that train and place service dogs and that subscribe to the high standards in training that are essential for the dogs' and humans' well being. ADI members also advocate for the acceptance and legitimacy of service dogs in mainstream society. ADI certifies and periodically re-certifies member training organizations to help ensure adherence to mandatory ADI standards. Sanitation of the facility, appropriate care and training of the dogs, adherence to applicable laws, and moral and reasonable treatment of clients are some of the categories in which ADI evaluates organizations for accreditation.[4]

If you are considering applying to a service dog placement agency, think with care—and with your future dog's best interests in mind—about what will happen if the program closes or changes to the point where support and follow-up from it are no longer available. This distressing situation happened to me when the San Francisco Society for the Prevention of Cruelty to Animals Hearing Dog Program (SF/SPCA HDP), an ADI-certified program, stopped without warning in April 2008. The SF/SPCA HDP had been a paragon for hearing dog programs for thirty years, and it had successfully placed about eight hundred shelter dogs (including Bogie) with Deaf and hard of hearing guardians who greatly benefited from these fantastic canine partners.

About three weeks after the sudden change, I and other SF/SPCA hearing dog guardians received a letter from the SF/SPCA informing us that a detailed examination of the HDP indicated that the program was no longer consistent with the mission of the organization. While the letter promised ongoing support for those of us who currently had hearing dogs from the SF/SPCA,[5] and a follow-up letter from the organization a month later offered to return applications on file to guardians requesting them (the letter also indicated that it would not keep a copy of a returned application; the applications contained a great deal of private information),[6] my trust in the organization and with the people running it dropped to less than zero.

My experience has taught me that new hearing dog applicants and current guardians should not take for granted the long-term stability of a hearing dog training center. Program certification, postplacement training, and follow-up commitments of a training organization are essential pieces of information to investigate and monitor, along with the vision of the organization's leaders. Here are a few points to keep in mind:

First, confirm privacy policies, security measures for your confidential information, and the use of all information that you give to an agency *before* you provide anything. While federal privacy laws protect your health information in many situations, as of this writing service dog agencies do not have to comply with Health Insurance Portability and Accountability Act regulations that doctors, hospitals, and other mainstream health care providers follow, so you will need to take a necessary leap of faith when you give a training agency your information.

Second, if you are accepted by a program and put on a waiting list, find out—in writing—what will happen if the program ends before you are placed with a dog. Does the program have a relationship with another organization that will be willing to add you to its waiting list? If so, are you willing to postpone getting a dog even longer? If not, will you be completely out of luck?

Third, consider your needs and expectations for ongoing support postplacement. Many guardians do not need a lot of brush-up training, but having a resource available will occasionally be helpful. Other guardians may benefit from frequent follow-up and training reinforcement. If a program ends, what will you do if you need assistance and cannot get it?

With those caveats in mind, though, remember that most service dog agencies are highly reputable and provide an outstanding service on behalf of dogs, guardians, and their communities. Approaching an agency in the spirit of cooperation can be the start of a rewarding partnership.

Public Access

Hearing dogs, along with all service dogs regardless of their functions, have public access rights throughout the United States. Federal and individual state laws ensure accessibility for specially trained service animals and provide penalties for interference with a service animal and noncompliance with statutes. Service dogs are permitted to accompany their human partners into restaurants and stores, to doctor and dentist appointments, and to sports and recreational venues. They are permitted on public transportation when accompanying their guardians, and they travel with their human partners in the passenger cabins on airplanes at no additional charge.

Dog licenses and vaccinations required of nonservice dogs are also mandatory for hearing dogs, although some local jurisdictions waive license fees for service dogs and issue special service dog license tags. While in public, a guardian is responsible for any damage caused by his hearing dog. Most training agencies issue a brightly colored cape and leash for each dog to wear to alert people that the dog is working and not to be disturbed. However, strangers often approach hearing dogs and try to pet them; guardians need to be firmly polite in letting others know that the dog is on duty.

The guardian must be willing to assume the responsibility of educating people about hearing dogs whenever he and his dog are out in public, and each of these situations presents an additional learning opportunity and bonding opportunity for the team to practice obedience in different circumstances.

Hearing Dog Illness, Retirement, and Passing

Occasionally during your dog's life he will get a minor illness or infection that will prevent him from doing his signal work for a few days. Rely on your veterinarian for advice about when your dog can resume his job; until then, let your canine partner take it easy. If your dog has a more serious injury—such as a broken limb—she may need several weeks or months of recuperation. Retraining for signal work, if your veterinarian and your dog's trainer are comfortable with your dog resuming signaling duties, may take a few more weeks. Be patient, and recommit to the training obligations that you assumed when you first partnered with your dog. She will probably be eager to get back into her routine.

At some point after you are partnered with a hearing dog, on what will be a very sad day, you will realize that your hearing dog needs to transition into retirement either because of an incurable illness or because of diminished hearing of his own. If you have received a hearing dog from a placement agency, the trainers will discuss transitioning to retirement with you during your initial training and in the years of follow up.

In general, your dog will stay with you for the duration of his life, becoming more of a pet during his later years. He will still respond to signals, though not as consistently as before, and your expectations of responsiveness will need to be lowered. Some training agencies will place another service dog with you while your retired hearing dog is still alive, but others will not. You may be more comfortable using assistive technology during this period, instead of introducing another dog into your home.

Throughout his life, your dog will be your partner, child, and best friend all rolled into one furry soul who depends on you as much as you depend on him. Not having him next to you will be treacherous and anguishing. When your dog dies, give yourself the time and space to mourn, and then to celebrate his life and the gifts he gave you every day. Friends and family can offer immeasurable support after a service dog dies, and you may also find that a pet-loss support group can help you transition into life without a canine partner; some resources are in appendix B. If you choose to get another service dog later on, you will know when the time is right.

The "Low-Tech" Advantage

Having a hearing dog can profoundly improve the quality of life of someone with a hearing loss. However a human gets information about the world—from one's ears, one's eyes, or a soft and furry paw—sound awareness is important, whether the person is awake or asleep, at home or at work, alone or with others.

Sophisticated hearing health care technology like powerful digital hearing aids and cochlear implants can turn silence into sound with the touch of a button. However, technology's usefulness as a social bonding mechanism is still constrained by its necessarily inanimate and insentient qualities. An attentive, responsive hearing dog is a remarkable and vibrant being who keeps his human partner glued to, and part of, the audible world with a most special, albeit intangible, social adhesive. This "low-tech" assistance can provide an immeasurable increase in comfort, security, and independence. The guardian will have a rare and important opportunity to nurture, love, and help another life thrive, while benefiting from an unparalleled relationship.

Tips for Living with a Hearing Service Dog

- If you are considering applying for a hearing dog, ask the training agency if you can spend a few hours with a hearing dog/guardian team to get a firsthand sense of what life will be like with a service animal.

- Before applying, make a list of sounds that are difficult for you to hear and find out if a hearing dog can be trained to help you. Some agencies will train hearing dogs for specially requested signals, but keep your expectations realistic; no hearing dog can be trained to respond to every sound that you have trouble hearing. Also, not all programs will train dogs to alert their guardians to some critical sounds such as a baby crying, because however well trained, the dogs will occasionally fail to respond for one reason or another.
- Make arrangements for your dog's care in case something happens to you. Some training agencies have policies for these situations, and others leave it up to the hearing dog recipient.
- Keep life quiet for the first few weeks after you are partnered with your new dog—everyone will want to meet him, but make introductions gradually to prevent overwhelming both of you with stressful new stimuli.
- Taking a hearing dog to work is manageable—stash poop bags in your jacket, in your desk, and even in your lunch bag. Keep a water bowl and extra treat rewards in your cube or office and plan frequent potty breaks. Prepare your co-workers before and after the arrival of your hearing dog with etiquette lessons.
- Do not bring a hearing dog to a place that contains obvious safety risks, such as an area of a health club where dumbbells can fall or a construction site where debris and extreme noise are hazards. Remember that you are aware of dangers that your dog will not know about unless he experiences them, and that you have the responsibility to anticipate risks for your dog.
- When traveling, always notify hotels, airlines, and car rental companies ahead of time that you have a service animal. While these businesses are required to provide access to service dogs, they don't like surprises, and many people think that service dogs are only for people who are blind or visually impaired. Send thank-you notes to managers of companies who treat you and your dog especially well.

- If you fly, get your dog used to the airport by having a few obedience practice sessions in the ticketing and baggage claim areas. Most airlines require that you get a health certificate from your veterinarian right before travel; many health certificates are only valid for ten days. Be sure to check the restrictions before you leave home to avoid having to get another certificate in your destination city in order to fly back. Travel to a rabies-free area (such as Hawaii or England) typically requires substantial documentation and advance planning to allow your service dog entry without quarantine.
- If people in your community ask you to give hearing dog demonstrations to their schools or organizations, agree to only as many as you feel comfortable doing. While increasing awareness about hearing dogs is important, your canine partner is trained to work with you in your life, not to perform. Demonstrations can be tiring for both you and your dog. Feel free to refer requests to your training agency; most are happy to arrange demonstrations with community groups.
- Remember that your dog is a dog first, and a service animal second. Love him fully, and cherish every day that you have together.

Flying the Furry Skies

Like many other people with a hearing loss, it can be hard for me to trust my ears. Having a pair of auditory antennae around that is so much better than my own is an important boost to my confidence, and it improves my ability to navigate everyday activities. There is also no substitute for having the opportunity to care for such a special canine.

Bogie is far too clever for his own good, but he possesses not an ounce of guile. He came into my life after I lost my first beloved hearing dog, Chelsey, to old age. Chelsey always had a thing for goldens, and I have a feeling that she sent Bogie to me. "The Boy," as I often think of him, and I graduated from the San Francisco SPCA Hearing Dog Program in June 2006, and he has been a sparkling, joyous presence in my life ever since.

Bogie is wicked smart, he learns effortlessly, and he is impressively efficient in alerting me. In the four-plus years since we became partners, he has amazed me over and over again with his responsiveness and signaling skills. No sound, however faint (or however unrelated it may be to his formal signal training) gets by Bogie—not so much as a bird chirping, a raindrop falling, or, most importantly, the treat bag rustling will fall below his übersensitive radar—and he loves his job as much as I love him.

A couple of years ago, when we took a plane trip from Sacramento to Seattle to visit John (then my fiancé), I saw—for the umpteenth time—just how competent Bogie really is. It all started when I was packing. While airport travel is a noisy headache for me, Bogie understands that suitcases mean lots of treats will be forthcoming; being patient in security lines, after all, has its rewards. A special day was coming up, and Bogie knew it. He was eager to get started, and he helped me pack his things by nudging them with his nose closer and closer to the backpack that I would wear on the plane. Health certificate from the vet, check. Chew toys, check. Collapsible water bowl, towel for mopping up spilled water (Bogie drinks with gusto, always), blankie, extra treats, doggie raincoat, emergency food, slicker brush and grooming rake—check-check-check-check-check-check-check-check.

Bogie loves to fly, but I have been paranoid about air travel since September 11, and those seat bottom flotation devices won't work for pooches. The Boy has a blaze-orange canine life preserver, so I tried it on him, made some adjustments, and packed his stylish-yet-functional accessory in the bottom compartment of my backpack. I hoped that we would never need it, and I said as much to the forces in the universe as I zipped up the backpack and tossed it into my car. I knew that I would have a similar chat with them shortly before takeoff the next day.

Bogie wakes me up every morning by nuzzling me with his nose—which is usually very cold and very wet—until I thank him and say good morning. A vibro-tactile alarm clock that I keep under my pillow triggers his wake-up service. It is indeed a brain-scrambling way to start the day, but to Bogie it means "treats" when it starts to shake and rattle.

If I show any resistance to getting up, such as lingering in bed for longer than five seconds—an eternity to a dog who has some 400,000 sounds and scents to catalog before the day is done— Bogie pulls the blankets off of me with his mouth and drags them to the floor. The steward of my consciousness at this early hour, Bogie knows his job well. He also knew that on this particular day the earlier he got me up and going, the sooner we would be on our way to the airport, and hence to the treat jackpot that is his edible salary. His wake-up motives are not entirely altruistic.

Not many people are fortunate enough to have a love-powered, fur-covered, sixty-five-pound alarm clock who never needs batteries. But this particular morning was one of those days when bed was just too comfortable, and I couldn't help but wish for a conventional snooze alarm that hearing people use to ease themselves into their days eight minutes at a time.

"Pulllleeeeze, Bog, just five more minutes, okay?" I croaked as I managed to open one eye to see that it was only 4:15 in the morning—much earlier than usual, because of our flight schedule—when Bogie shocked me out of sleep with his nose and several slobbery canine kisses. I thought that I could dawdle just a little before hauling myself back into the world of the living. I tried to pull the blankets over my head to dry my face, but Bogie took my burrowing as a game, and I could feel him growling playfully while he pulled the covers off of the bed. He plopped onto my torso, informing me with his eager pant and relentlessly whipping tail that, "Hey, if I can wake up early, so can you. Oh, and by the way, you owe me a treat." I sighed, moved his strong paws off of my shoulders, gave him a treat from my stash in the nightstand, and shuffled to my feet.

I needed to hustle to get myself together and put on my hearing aids so that I could rejoin the hearing world and get to the airport on time. While I got ready, Bogie, his first task of the morning completed, began to practice his canine yoga—"Boga" I call it (the bow; the full-body back stretch; and, to end his routine, what I think of as the catapult pose, his graceful body extended to nearly five feet on the rug, his hips turned out so far that Rudolf Nureyev would have been impressed, and his rear paws assumed a poised-and-ready-to-spring position). After a brief period of contemplation, during which Bogie was no doubt mulling over what was for breakfast and how long he was going to have to wait for it, The Boy jumped to all fours and trotted to the kitchen. We ate breakfast (well, more accurately, I ate; he vacuumed) in record time, and then headed out to the airport.

Bogie got more and more excited as we approached the terminal, and we went into what I call "movie star mode" the moment we got out of the car. Everyone—and I mean everyone—turned to stare at Bogie as we made our way to the check-in line; head after head after head followed Bogie's golden coat and happy-go-lucky demeanor all the way to the baggage counter. Some people smiled, some stared with open jaws, some pointed, and a few looked stunned. I was glad that I'd thrown on some makeup, because people were staring at me as if I were walking next to an Oscar winner or a tabloid headliner, neither of whom could command as much attention as a hearing dog does in an airport. That people ever look at *me* is a grand delusion on my part. I am merely the invisible human on the other end of the leash, and I am well aware of my transparency. It's all about the dog, folks.

The litany of stock questions and reactions, which I know by heart, started while we were waiting in line to check our suitcases.

"Is that a guide dog?" a man wearing earbuds and portable music player asked. He spoke loudly—even by my standards—so I gathered that whatever he was listening to was cranked up pretty high.

"No," I replied, "he's a hearing service dog. I am deaf without my hearing aids, and my dog hears for me," I explained.

"What?" the man asked. "It's hard to hear you in here."

I gestured to my ear hardware and turned my head so that the man could see it. (By the way, don't believe any hearing aid dispenser who tells you that other people will think that hearing aids look like James Bond-ish, hands-free cell phone receivers. People often stare at the aids, and me, with horror and chagrin.) "No, he's a *hearing dog*," I said slowly and emphatically.

The man stared at my ear hardware, got that "ewwww" expression on his face that I have seen thousands of times, and walked away. I shrugged, Bogie wagged his tail, and we inched forward in the line. A moment later, two school-age girls rushed up to Bogie, waving their hands in his face and giggling, and nearly startling him out of his down-stay. I scratched his ears to help him relax.

"Hey, kids," I said, "My dog is working, so I'd appreciate it if you wouldn't pet him. He needs to stay focused."

"We just wanted to say hello," one of the girls said. She tried to pull Bogie's tail, so I told Bogie to move behind me, and I gave him another few treats. He was only too happy to oblige.

"I know," I answered, "But this is a service animal. You need to stay away from him." I was more forceful this time, and I could feel my face assuming its "this-is-what-I-look-like-when-I'm-walking-on-the-streets-of-New-York" expression. In other words, don't mess with me and stay away from my dog.

"You're not very nice," the other girl said with a huffy scowl, as they both backed away. I saw them eventually find the adults whom I assume were their parents; the kids chattered to the adults while gesturing towards me, and one of the grown-ups gave me a withering glare that would curdle vanilla ice cream. However tempting it was for me to march over there and have a chat with them about service animals, this was turning into one of those leave-it-alone moments. I turned away and checked the flight departure monitor as the check-in line crept forward. Bogie, however, kept his eyes on those kids; he didn't want to be bum-rushed again.

When Bogie and I were at the front of the line, I felt a tap on my shoulder.

"Excuse me," an elderly lady said from the row behind us in the serpentine. "Your dog is beautiful. How old is she, or is she a he?" she inquired, while not-so-surreptitiously sneaking a peek at Bogie's underside.

"Thank you," I responded with a laugh. "He is about three, and definitely male."

The lady nodded. "Oh, that's a fun age. When I got divorced, I adopted a kitty-cat who was three, and I had her for fifteen years. My goodness, did she shed! Her name was Emma. And my ex-husband and I had two yellow labs who were brother and sister, and they mated but the interbreeding caused some birth defects in the puppies and it was a very. . . ."

"Sorry, we've got to go," I interjected. I added a hasty "nice talking to you" before I looked away. It seems like at least one person in an airport line always wants to tell me his or her life story, and it's not that I'm uninterested or that I don't care, but trying to carry on a conversation amidst the hubbub, with a big dog on one side of me and more than one hundred pounds of luggage on the other side, takes all of my concentration. More than once I have missed seeing a baggage representative wave me over to the check-in counter; the person who was directly behind me in line the last time that happened actually shoved me forward because he was in such a hurry. My mission on this day was to arrive in Seattle without sporting a broken nose and to be able to greet John in one piece.

After all of that excitement, checking in was a breeze. The agent matched Bogie's service dog ID card—in his photograph, he is, I swear, smiling—to his health certificate and gave me the baggage claim checks. Most travelers at this point would be on their way to security, but those of us with service dogs have to head outside one last time for the requisite preflight potty break.

Few airports have dedicated dog areas, but out of about fifteen airports into which Bogie (and Chelsey, in years past) and I have flown, we have always managed to find a place for a break. We have had several mini-adventures in the process. At the Pittsburgh International Airport we had to take a tram from the terminal and almost missed our connecting flight; at O'Hare in Chicago we landed in subzero temperatures and Chelsey learned about snow during our layover; and at Malpensa Airport in Milan, Italy, there were acres and acres of fields just right for preflight canine frolicking and sniffing. And always, countless stares, smiles, waves, and laughs from passersby greeted us.

One summer several years ago, Chelsey and I even met a Good Samaritan. We had to change planes early in the morning at Sky Harbor International Airport in Phoenix, but because of a delay before the second leg of our flight we had some extra time to wander around outside. Arizona in summer is gloriously bright even before the desert heat kicks in, and I was wearing oversized sunglasses when Chelsey—wearing her service dog cape, as usual—and I walked out of the terminal. I saw a patch of manicured lawn across the traffic lanes, and as we waited for the crosswalk light to change, a kind lady put her hand on my shoulder and said in a loud, deliberate voice, "Honey, the terminal is behind you, but don't you worry—I'll help you and your dog back inside."

I turned to the woman with a flummoxed expression on my face until I realized a second later that she thought that I was blind. I got a big smile on my face, pushed my sunglasses to the top of my head, gestured to my ears, and said, "Oh, thank you, but I can see. I am hearing impaired, and this is my hearing service dog. We are just going across the street for a bathroom break." Chelsey thumped her tail in greeting.

"Oh, how wonderful for you," the lady said, very, very loudly. "Do you need any help?"

"Thank you, I think we'll be fine," I responded, coughing back a laugh, "but I appreciate your asking. I really am grateful for your kindness."

"All righty," she said with an exaggerated wave as she turned away. I waved back, with a lighter feeling inside than I'd had a minute before. The episode was funny, but heartwarming too. For the rest of our brief stay in Phoenix, I made a point to wave to people who were looking at us so that they would know that I could see. They probably thought that I was nuts, but that happens a lot anyway.

Back in Sacramento, Bogie made a beeline for the spacious lawns about a quarter of a mile from the terminal, where he has chased squirrels and let out preflight steam many times. We circled around his favorite tree area three times while Bogie inspected thousands of blades of grass, and then headed back to the terminal.

At last we were on our way to security. The insanely long line leading to the checkpoint stretched almost out to the parking garage entrance. Now patience is not one of my virtues. My wonderful dog is teaching me, though, a little bit each day, about cultivating serenity from within when we don't have any other choice. We made slow progress through the maze that led to the metal detector, and over the next half hour or so Bogie scored a treat every few minutes from the pouch that I had clipped around my waist for being an absolute gentleman in line. Step, step, step, wait; down-stay, treat. Repeat. People in this security line were somber—probably because there were several military personnel nearby, armed with very big guns—and everyone waiting to go through security watched Bogie admiringly and respectfully.

In case you're wondering—and, well, even if you're not—hearing dogs have to be cleared through security just like us humans. When we got to the screening area I took off Bogie's cape, collar (with five tags, the accessory qualifies as "canine bling"), and leash and put them in a tray for scanning in the X-ray machine. The first time Bogie had to undress in the airport, he seemed a bit embarrassed by his nakedness, but he's comfortable preparing for his strip search now (and better him than me, however selfish that may sound).

We went through the metal detector single file. I gave Bogie his down-stay command before I walked through the detector—Bogie focused on me with laser-like precision—and then I called him to me. A Transportation Security Administration (TSA) guard asked Bogie to sit for his physical examination; the guard ran his fingers through The Boy's fur and examined inside his ears, under his tail, and in between his toes, checking for contraband. Bogie sat patiently during the search, and he gave the guard a big smooch when it was over. If I had done such a thing, I probably would have gotten arrested.

I was putting Bogie's uniform back on when another TSA officer, who was holding my backpack, waved me over to the hand-search area. His expression was somber.

"Excuse me, ma'am, is there anything in here that can hurt me?" he asked.

I was baffled. "No, I don't think so," I said blankly.

"Do you mind if I search through your belongings?" the guard queried.

"No, of course I don't mind," I squeaked, as I wondered if I was about to be hauled off to jail. (What did I do? What did I do?)

"There is something in here that resembles a gun according to the X-ray machine," the TSA officer said sternly, as he started unzipping the compartments of my backpack in a very practiced and efficient manner. I am not known for packing lightly, so all kinds of sundry stuff, ranging from gum to lip gloss to my pocket calculator—oh, *that's* where I put it—started spilling out onto the examination table. "Do you know what it could be?" he asked.

I lifted my shoulders and eyebrows and held all four of them as high as my ears in genuine bewilderment. I could feel my eyes get big and my heart pounding close to my throat. Getting stopped for a speeding ticket is less terrifying than going through airport security these days. Visions of a bunch of National Guardsmen converging around me and pointing AK-47 guns in my face in a matter of seconds whizzed through my mind.

"I-I-I really don't know, sir," I stammered. I started prattling off all of the essentials that I had crammed into my pack for the ninety-minute flight. "I've got a couple of king-size candy bars, but neither is as big as a gun, and some crackers and my data files and makeup and pens and my journal and a deck of cards and a couple of books and a first-aid kit and a package of tissues and a bag of trail mix and my camera and my dog's portable water bowl and his treats and his toys—*oh!*—there's a big hard chewy bone in there for my dog that might be what you saw. Could that be it?" I asked.

The guard rummaged through the rest of my things and found Bogie's bone. He handed it to the examiner at the X-ray machine, at which point Bogie, who had been waiting nonchalantly, instantly became interested in the situation. Someone else had one of his prized possessions, and The Boy can indeed be possessive when it comes to his toys. He remained in his down-stay position, but his chocolate-brown eyes unblinkingly followed his bone as the second guard scrutinized all sides of it, saw the telltale fang marks on it, nodded, and gave it back to the first guard.

"This object has been cleared," the first TSA guard said, as he handed the object of everyone's interest back to me. "You can proceed to your flight."

My shoulders and eyebrows dropped instantly, as did my blood pressure. "Thank you," I replied with a deep exhale. Bogie also heaved a relieved sigh and thump-thump-thumped his tail on the floor when I put the bone back in my pack, and I made a mental note to take the bone out for a separate inspection on our return flight. Every day with a hearing dog is a learning experience!

Because of the bone-induced delay in getting through security, Bogie and I had to race over to the gate where our flight was already boarding. Passengers with service animals get to preboard, so we squeezed in at the front of the line. Interestingly, most passengers have been pretty understanding about dogs on planes since September 11. Even though Bogie is not an explosives-detection dog (he would almost certainly ferret out stray peanuts and pretzel crumbs on the floor of a plane cabin before he found a bomb), it seems as if passengers just feel more comfortable having dogs on flights these days. Chelsey and I had gotten more than our share of slit-eyed stares and nasty comments when we first started flying together in the mid-1990s, but tolerance levels are a lot higher now.

On the plane at last, I settled into the bulkhead window seat, which gives Bogie more room on the floor than in a regular row. The flight attendants all asked to meet Bogie, and he was a gracious passenger, shaking paws with everyone and loving the attention. Crew members are always crazy about him; when the time comes for the emergency demonstration prior to takeoff, Bogie is pretty much the only one paying attention. He watches raptly as flight attendants use hand signals to point out the locations of the emergency exits and the oxygen masks, and they seem grateful to have an audience.

I have never told them that the reason Bogie is so interested in their instructions is because many of the hand signals that they use are similar to the signs that Bogie learned in his hearing dog training. They think that he just likes to watch them do their jobs, and I have been smart enough—well, until now—to maintain the fiction. It makes for better public relations all the way around.

Before we took off, I gave Bogie some ice cubes to chew on while we were ascending. The chewing helps to relieve air pressure in his ears, in the same way that chewing gum helps humans keep their ears clear during changes in altitude. He chomped happily as the plane headed off to Seattle, and I settled down to write in my journal.

The flight itself was relatively uneventful. The other human passenger sitting in our row was busy watching a DVD, and I was happy to have the luxury of an hour and a half of relative tranquility. While I have met some fascinating people on airplanes, a couple of times, and I am only a little ashamed to admit this, I have turned off my hearing aids or speech processor so that I didn't have to listen to a chatty seatmate or to a baby crying for hours on end. Once we reached cruising altitude, Bogie sacked out for a well-earned nap, though his ears perked up whenever a crew member made an announcement. I don't hear those, but I can usually tell from the context of everyone's behavior what is happening, whether it's unexpected turbulence making people buckle up or the final approach to landing necessitating raising the seatbacks.

This landing was a little on the bumpy side, and we could see that it was raining hard in Seattle. Bogie looked out the window with anticipation as we taxied to the gate; he was happy that we were back on terra firma. When the plane parked, Bogie and I said good-bye to the flight crew, and we walked briskly down to the main terminal where John was waiting with open arms to hug both Bogie and me, and then all of us headed to baggage claim.

Bogie and I zipped outside for his postflight potty break while John waited for our luggage, and on our way back in, we saw two preschoolers playing on the floor next to the baggage carousel. Bogie kept a wary eye on them, but he seemed to sense that they were different from the obnoxious kids we had seen earlier. These youngsters were content to throw crayons at each other and pull each other's hair, and to leave Bogie alone. Their mother looked at Bogie while she pulled her kids apart and she said to me, "Your dog is beautiful, and so well behaved!"

I replied with a smile, "Thank you. Your kids are great too."

She looked incredulous. One of her offspring had just thrown a handful of wood blocks into the air, while the other shrieked, "I'm telling!!" I was grateful for the compression feature in my electronic ears.

"Wanna trade?" the mother asked, with a tortured expression that seemed only half-joking.

I chuckled. "Nope. But thanks for asking. And your kids will grow up, you know. My guy will be a kid forever."

As if on cue, Bogie did a happy wiggle on the floor in affirmation and celebration of his eternal puppyhood. I gave The Boy a treat. The world was just as it should be.

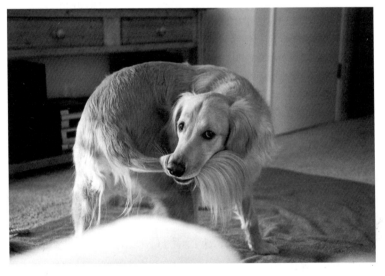

Bogie at play—even working dogs chase their tails! Photo credit: © 2008 John S. Batinovich. All rights reserved.

8

Learning for a Lifetime: Continuing Education and Career Growth

PEOPLE WITH HEARING loss can fully participate in higher education with a little planning and a flexible mindset, and they can compete successfully with students who do not have any hearing loss. Continuing education, professional development, and degree programs pursued part-time while on the job can add to a worker's sense of self-worth, increase a worker's value to an employer, and improve overall life satisfaction.

This chapter begins with an overview of educational attainment among working-age people and examines the disparities between those with and without hearing loss. Ways to learn in both traditional and 21st-century settings follow, along with some helpful listening strategies. The author's experiences with discrimination in education then show the importance of self-advocacy. The chapter concludes with lighter anecdotes that illustrate the humorous side of getting an education with a hearing loss.

Educational Attainment and Hearing Loss

Research shows that hearing loss can be a barrier to educational attainment. As seen in figure 19, almost half—48 percent—of working-age people over 25 years old with moderate or a lot of trouble hearing do not go onto college and the percentage of people earning at least a bachelor's degree decreases as the severity of hearing loss increases. About one-third—32 percent—of people with excellent or good hearing have earned a college degree, while 27 percent of people with a little trouble hearing and 24 percent of people with moderate or a lot of trouble hearing have attained this level of education.

Although people with hearing loss are less likely to graduate from college, those who do graduate have earning potentials similar to those without hearing loss. According to the 2008 National Health Interview Survey, among people in the working-age group who are at least 25 years old and have any trouble hearing,

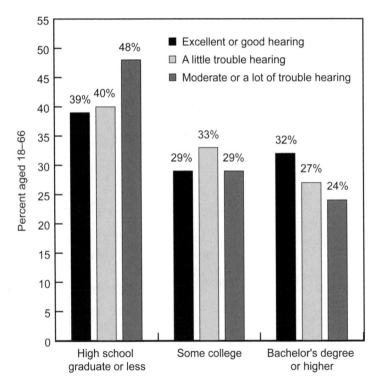

Figure 19. Educational attainment among the working-age group over 25 years old by hearing category, United States, 2008. *High school graduates include people who have earned GEDs. Analysis includes working-age respondents ages 26–66 and excludes refused to answer, not ascertained, and don't know responses.*

59 percent with a bachelor's degree or higher earned $45,000 or more in 2007. Among people in this age group who have excellent or good hearing, 60 percent with a bachelor's degree or higher earned at least $45,000 in the same year.[1]

The direct relationship between education and earnings is well known. In general, the more education a person has, the more money she or he makes over her or his working life. The Census Bureau has reported that "full-time, year-round workers with a bachelor's degree" had annual earned income 1.8 times higher than people with a high school diploma in 1999, and workers with a master's, professional, or doctoral degree earned 2.6 times as much as high school graduates in the same year.[2]

More education may help to increase your work income. Many workers can take advantage of financial assistance—some employers offer tuition reimbursement to employees who earn good grades in courses related to their jobs, for example, and the Federal Lifetime Learning Credit can save you money on your taxes when you take qualified courses. Appendix B contains links to more information about tax benefits for education.

Learning Options

More options than ever before exist for people already in the labor force to enhance their skills, regardless of hearing ability. Traditional classes, online (distance) learning, and telecourses are three ways that you can build your skill set and enrich your knowledge.

Traditional Classes

If you enjoy interacting with other students and have convenient access to a four-year or a community college, going to school in a bricks-and-mortar setting could be your best option. Check the newspaper or online catalogs of your local schools for courses or degree programs that interest you; many schools also have open houses and career fair days that you can attend to get information about classes. Then, make an appointment with a counselor in the advising office to discuss your goals and the accommodations available to students with hearing disabilities. If you are interested in earning a degree, map out a realistic timeline with your advisor. It may take several years to finish your program, but the investment will be well worth the effort and an achievement of which you, your family, and your friends will be very proud.

If you are older than most college students, let your age work to your advantage. You will find that professors love "re-entries" (older students who have taken a break from college) because they are often more motivated to learn and more engaged with their studies than their younger counterparts. You will probably enjoy the energy that comes from being around such a diverse group and may find that you learn as much from your junior academic colleagues as you do from your peers at work.

When I went back to school, I was 28 and had just been fitted with my first pair of hearing aids. I was working three jobs at the time—one full-time and two part-time—and so was able to take just one class, one night a week. (I thought that I would be in school forever!) My course load increased a little bit each year as scholarship assistance enabled me to scale back work, and I finished my bachelor's degree when I was 34. Never once did I feel out of place, old, or unwelcome. On the contrary, I had a blast going to school with some people who were half a lifetime younger than I, and I thrived in the collegiate setting.

To help you explore your options, most schools will allow you to sit in on some lectures to get a sense of course material firsthand. You can take a tour of the campus from a student guide who will give you a frontline perspective on the campus culture. Community colleges offer both academic and vocational classes with tuition and fees much lower than costs at traditional four-year institutions, and class sizes are usually much smaller. The credit for many classes can transfer to universities offering bachelor's degrees.

Saturday-only classes, evening degree and extension programs, short courses, and intersession "boot camps" offered between regular terms are alternatives to full-time day classes. These give you the ability to participate in college life, work toward a degree, and enhance your professional skills while working and taking care of family responsibilities. These choices also let you try out different subjects and learning environments with a smaller investment of your time.

Online Classes

You can't beat the Internet for convenient learning around the clock, with little to no demands on your hearing. Just about every college offers "distance learning" from the comfort of your own home in dozens of different subjects ranging from art history to zoology. If you have the discipline to pace yourself throughout the term and like to work independently, distance learning can be a fantastic way to build your skill set without taxing your ears. Keep in mind that course grades for online work go on a transcript just like grades from classes taken in a traditional academic setting do, and it can be very easy to forget about assignment due dates and course withdrawal deadlines when you are not heading to campus on a regular basis. Transcripts do not expire, so your grades will follow you forever.

Online coursework offered for degree credit or a certificate program sometimes entails an introductory in-person meeting, and it usually requires assignments that you e-mail to the instructor throughout the course. If you plan to transfer credit or apply coursework to a degree, make sure that the institution offering the course is accredited—some online "schools" churn out paper-mill degrees or certificates that will not help you academically or professionally, regardless of the price that you pay for them. The U.S. Department of Education maintains a database of accredited colleges and programs that you can access online; see appendix B for the source.

Telecourses

Community colleges also offer distance learning classes via community television broadcasts. Registration is done at the community college—either in-person or through an online system—and communication with the course instructor is through e-mail with occasional in-person meetings. Course content includes both academic subjects, such as Shakespearean drama, and vocational or personal enrichment topics, such as winemaking.

Telecourse program "assignments" usually air two or three times during the week listed on the course syllabus. Students complete homework assignments or problem sets relating to the weekly shows and then e-mail their work to the instructor for grading. Some supplemental reading may be required, with books available either at the campus bookstore or online.

The most important issue for a telecourse student with a hearing loss is whether or not the programs are closed-captioned. While almost all programming is required to be captioned, be sure to confirm with an e-mail to the instructor that all of the required course programs are accessible to you. Do not leave captioning—or any other accommodations—to chance.

Participating in College with a Hearing Loss

Plenty of resources for managing your hearing loss in school are available, but you will need to take the first step. Both the Americans with Disabilities Act of 1990 (with amendments) and the Rehabilitation Act of 1973 mandate the accessibility of educational institutions that receive federal funding. What makes a course or a campus accessible to an individual varies by the disability and by the student. In postsecondary (after high school) educational settings, the responsibility for requesting reasonable accommodations for your hearing loss is yours alone.

The school must have a process for you to follow to request and obtain what you need, and schools need to have qualified personnel available to assess what will work best for you, to provide accommodations in working order and on time, and to enforce campus compliance with disability laws. You can initiate the process by contacting the disabled students' office on your campus as soon as you have decided to attend school or at the latest when you register for classes. If you register late or add a class after a term starts, the school must still provide reasonable accommodations.

People with hearing loss are entitled to several kinds of accommodations, including note-takers, real-time captioning, FM and infrared loop systems (also called assistive listening devices or ALDs) in auditoriums and large lecture halls, and front-row seating (see chapter 1 for a description of these accommodations). Some Deaf and hard of hearing people request sign language interpreters. If an instructor uploads live lectures to the Internet as part of a traditional or an online course, the school will need to caption these talks or make a transcript available. It is a good idea to check with the instructor before registering for such a course, so that she or he can make the necessary arrangements for any spoken material to be accessible to everyone.

What is considered "reasonable" by a school's disability staff may not be what you want—you may, for example, prefer real-time captioning for a lecture that is scheduled in a hall that has a loop system—but the school has satisfied the law if the accommodation is appropriate for the situation. An instance where an accommodation would not be reasonable is if a sign language interpreter were arranged for a student who does not sign.

A quick comment about note-takers—try to work with a note-taker who has a writing style close enough to your own to make the notes useful. Note-takers are usually fellow students in each of your lecture classes who are academically strong with regular attendance records and who are able to take clear notes of all material, including questions posed by other students during each class meeting. This accommodation is most useful in lectures and least useful in discussion groups. Your school's disabled students' office will assign a note-taker, and his or her notes will supplement your own, but not replace them. If after the first lecture you are not able to extract useful information from your note-taker's pages, meet with her or him outside of class to clarify what will work for you before the term progresses any further.

A Few Potential Obstacles, and Workarounds that Work

As a student with a hearing loss, you may encounter some challenges in managing your disability, including not hearing some lecture material, managing the borrowing and returning of campus assistive listening equipment, "hearing" films that are not captioned, studying in a group, and hearing proctors during entrance exams and placement tests. The suggestions that follow can help you clear these hurdles.

Missing What Is Said in Class

Bluff not, or thou shalt be bluffed! If you miss some information in class, meet with the professor during office hours or send an e-mail to fill in the gaps. Be brief and to the point, and do not expect preferential treatment or a free pass because you did not hear something.

Accommodation Logistics

Schools vary in their policies about listening devices; some will let you use one for an entire term, and others require you to check out and return the equipment each day so that other students can use it. Always return the device and its accessories on time. More than a common courtesy, if you do not comply with the rules for borrowing equipment, you may have student privileges and services revoked, including library use and the ability to register for future classes.

Allow enough time before class for you and your professor to set up and test an ALD, and sufficient time after the class to collect the equipment. Some professors habitually run late, and are so busy talking during a class period that they will not remember that you (and other students) have other commitments right after their lectures end. You may need to be assertive in reminding some of your teachers that you need your device back. If you can, space out your classes so that you have breaks between them.

Films that Are Not Captioned

While almost all new productions are captioned, once in a while an older film or documentary will part of a course's required content and captioning the one copy on short notice may not be feasible for your school. When that happened to me in a rhetoric class at the University of California, Berkeley, in 1996, I was worried about not being able to understand the dialogue in the movie. When I brought up the situation to my professor, he was not worried at all. He had a copy of the script, and he lent it to me so that I could follow the film with everyone else in class and not miss a word. It was a terrific solution. Libraries and drama and film departments on most campuses have scripts of thousands of plays and movies, so check those sources if your professor does not have a copy.

Study Groups

Most of the time, background noise is the problem when you are preparing for an exam with your fellow students. Try to reserve a room in the library instead of meeting in a clattering coffeehouse off campus. Keep the lighting bright and sit with your back to any windows. Be an asset to your study group, not a liability—be prepared, be on time, and be ready to contribute at least your share to the discussion. If you need a listening device for the group, make arrangements at least a week ahead of time to pick one up from your disabled students' center.

Entrance Exams and Placement Tests

Whether required by your school or a future graduate or professional program, at some point in your academic lifetime you will probably have to take a sit-down exam such as a math placement test to determine the right class for you after admission, or a graduate test requirement such as Graduate Record Examination (GRE). The organizations that administer these tests are required to provide reasonable accommodations, and they should have published policies for requesting what you need. Follow these policies exactly, keep written documentation of all correspondence, and confirm arrangements a week before the exam date.

Get the contact information for the proctor or test center manager who will be on-site the day of your exam. A central office manages registration for most major tests such as the GRE, but the exams are administered at hundreds of locations. You need to have someone available at your particular testing site who is experienced in providing accommodations for a hearing loss and who will be responsible for any problems you may encounter with them, such as dead batteries in an ALD. Be sure to get approval for these accommodations well before the testing date.

When I registered for the pencil-and-paper version of the GRE in 1996, I made arrangements with the Educational Testing Service (ETS) main office in Princeton, New Jersey, for an ALD at the testing site in San Francisco well in advance of the test date. When I arrived at the exam location an hour ahead of time, nobody there knew anything about an ALD. One of the proctors sent me on a wild goose chase, and another shunted me off into a room of dental exam students. When I finally got to the right room about two minutes before the test started, no ALD was available, and the proctor was clueless about it. I could not hear anything the proctor was saying to anyone in the room.

I wanted to scream in exasperation, but I took the exam instead. I had practiced for it, and I had to take it. Whether or not I missed vital spoken information remains a mystery; my mindset at that point was to do the best I could and move on. By the time I finished the exam, I was both stressed and angry.

A few weeks later—after I got my scores—I complained to ETS with the assistance of the California Center for Law & the Deaf (an advocacy organization that unfortunately closed in 2008), and several months later, ETS refunded my testing fee. The organization did not admit any wrongdoing, and I never did find out who or what department messed up so thoroughly, or why. And as for my scores, they wound up being competitive enough, so I was happy that I had taken the exam. Would my numbers have been higher if I had had the amplification that I needed and if I had been less tense because of the testing staff ignorance? Probably, but I am glad that I did not give up and walk away. I was off to grad school!

A Heinous Example of Discrimination

I still remember my excitement when I received an offer of admission to the master's program in communication studies at the University of North Carolina in Chapel Hill (UNC) in 1997. That program was my top choice, and my two visits to the campus before moving out there from California had been quite positive. I had met with several professors who had research interests that meshed well with mine, the other students in the department were super smart and friendly, and the campus itself was beautiful.

During both of my visits I talked to staff in the disabled students' office, and the interim director assured me that the campus was equipped to accommodate students with hearing loss. I expected no less from a five-star research-university. My audiologist sent verification of my hearing loss several months before my classes started, and I was confident that I would have a hassle-free two years in the Southeast as far as my ears were concerned.

I was wrong. Even before class started, I began to notice serious problems on campus. When I tried to arrange accommodations for a required teaching assistant workshop before the fall semester began, the interim disability services director gave me incorrect information about the compatibility of an auditorium's public address system with my own ALD, and he did not follow up with me as promised when I told him about the problem. During the workshop, I could hear next to nothing. I tried to piece together what people were saying from context and the bits and pieces that I did understand, but I left the event feeling confused and worn out.

A few weeks later the interim director told me that the campus did not have the listening equipment available and that there were neither written records of equipment for hearing loss, nor procedures for getting what I needed. The interim director told me that I was not supposed to try to get accommodations on my own because some people on campus considered people with disabilities to be a bother.

It is rare for me to feel helpless, but after that directive and the workshop debacle, I had no confidence in the UNC disability services staff to provide reasonable accommodations to me, to communicate effectively with me, or to comply with the law regarding services to students with verified disabilities. That meeting set off a series of conferences and e-mails with my department chair and my faculty advisor—both of whom unequivocally supported my position—and led to my sitting down with the campus's vice chancellor for student services to discuss the problems I had experienced with the disabled students' office and my utter frustration at missing so much material in my courses.

At that appointment, I again requested the accommodations that I needed so that I could hear and participate in class—such as real-time captioning—and the vice chancellor wrote them down. I also told the vice chancellor that I wanted some clear answers about available accommodations and the procedures for getting them within two weeks. The semester had started a few weeks earlier, and the difficulty that I was having in my classes and discussion groups had gotten to the point where going to class was an exercise in futility. I was not able to follow the back-and-forth exchanges that characterized an academic program for someone majoring in communications and specializing in disability research. The contradiction was not lost on me.

What the disability services office sent me a couple of weeks later was a packet of generic information that had no relevance to my situation, such as captioned televisions in the dorms, and a form for requesting an interpreter. UNC never addressed my specific requests, nor did the university provide me with procedures to follow for getting equipment or captioning that I needed. By that point I had no confidence in UNC's intentions to accommodate my requests, which were reasonable. If the designated people at UNC had done their jobs, they could have provided my accommodations efficiently and at little cost.

While my fellow students and my professors were supportive, instances occurred on campus where I was treated horribly. In the library, for example, one of the student employees shouted at me that I was not allowed to bring my hearing service dog into the building. North Carolina is one of the few states to require service animal certification, so I showed the clerk Chelsey's state-issued service dog card, which had a photo of both of us on it. The employee had never heard of a hearing dog, and he nastily, and loudly, told me to get out and to take Chelsey with me.

I ignored him after that (I have never been one to be intimidated by what a friend of mine calls "self-appointed whatevers"), and I went to a librarian and showed her Chelsey's card. I told her that I was a grad student and that I had work to do, and if she had a problem with that, to call the campus police. Whether or not she did, I do not know, but except for some dirty looks, the library staff left us alone from that point. When Chels and I left the library a couple of hours later, I did not even glance at the staff members behind the circulation desk.

When the interim disability director dropped the ball again a few days later, this time not following up as promised to have me test a piece of equipment that might have worked for me, I decided that there was no point in continuing to spend massive amounts of my time and energy on an intractable situation. I went to UNC to be a grad student and yet was unable to participate in class.

My first semester was already half over, and each day had been full of pointlessness and aggravation. I was not sleeping; I was sad and confused; I felt like I could trust no one on campus; and I was spending more of my waking hours writing e-mails and meeting with faculty and staff to address accommodations issues than studying. I was not able to do what I had come to UNC to do, and I had no reason to believe (and I had several reasons to not believe) that my situation would improve. My faculty advisor and department chair—both tenured professors and highly respected on campus—were not able to get the disabled students' staff and leadership to do their jobs, either.

On October 9, 1997, I withdrew from UNC. It was an agonizing decision, but the right one under the circumstances. Several people on campus were dismayed, and a reporter for the student paper, The Daily Tar Heel, interviewed me about my withdrawal for a story later that month. The article summarized my position with my quote, "If I had been given accurate information, I never would have even applied to UNC."[3] I was hoping that I would be able to enroll at another school that was compliant with disability laws, and at which I could participate without restriction. But in the immediate future, all I wanted to do was end the UNC chapter of my life and try to move forward.

That plan also went awry. While I was packing for my move from Chapel Hill back to California I received a bill from UNC for $3,379.03 with no explanation for the amount due. I went to the cashier's office on campus to find what was going on, because when I withdrew, I had a zero balance with the university. My withdrawal would not have been processed if I had had so much as a library overdue fine on my account.

The cashier told me that my fellowship, which had paid the bulk of my tuition before I withdrew, was rescinded retroactively right after I withdrew without notice to me. Since I had attended classes at UNC, I owed the full amount. Also, the cashier informed me that, because tuition was due the previous July and it was now November, my account was seriously past due even though that was not yet reflected on my bill, and my account could be sent to a collection agency if I did not pay the full amount immediately. She did a good job scaring me, and I don't scare easily.

As people who know me well can tell you, it also takes a lot to render me irate, but wow, this situation did it. I was also speechless for about a minute as my body absorbed what was going on. I could feel rage gripping my jaw, making my knees lock, my stomach harden, my breath become shallow and my eyes narrow into slits. What do you do in such a circumstance? The cashier, of course, was merely being paid to do a job and not to think with even a modicum of common sense. Shouting at her would have done no good. With the threat of collection activity and its consequent destruction of my credit rating looming over my head, I paid the bill out of my savings and got a dated receipt before I left the cashier's office. I stomped back to my car and snarled at everybody I saw on the drive back to my apartment.

Chelsey and I took a long, long walk after that, while I mulled over my options. Letting this whole situation go was not something I would consider anymore. The discrimination, the denial of my education, and the financial manipulation had transgressed my threshold for shenanigans. When I told my relatives and friends about the cashier's bombshell, everyone was almost as galled as I was; several suggested taking legal action. The Internet led me to the Office for Civil Rights (OCR), which is responsible for enforcing disability laws at institutions that receive monies from the U.S. Department of Education.

I cooled off for a few days before filing a complaint with OCR, and then I started looking for an attorney. The prospect of initiating a lawsuit did not thrill me. I come from a family with its share of civil litigators, and I know how draining and tense any legal proceeding can be. My father, who had passed away several years before, was a lawyer who always championed the underdog. Whenever I had doubts about proceeding with the lawsuit, I remembered his sage words from my childhood: "Princess, be crazy when you need to be, and you'll be fine." But I also knew from my reading about OCR activity that while the agency could address the discriminatory treatment to which I had been subjected at UNC, it was unlikely that OCR would be able to get my money back for me. I would not tolerate what I saw as UNC making me pay them to discriminate against me.

Trying to find a lawyer willing to represent me was a task that started in November 1997 and lasted until after I returned to California the following month. Not one single attorney I approached who practiced in Chapel Hill was willing to even consider taking my case; two of them flat-out told me that I did not have a chance of being successful fighting UNC. Their words made me even more determined to try to right the wrongs. One of the property managers at my apartment complex, who had been enormously supportive since my access problems had started on campus over the summer, suggested that I try looking for a lawyer in nearby Durham—home to archrival Duke University. "Go to Duke, Sara," she urged. "They hate UNC over there!"

It was good advice. A referral from a law office in Durham led me to Patterson, Harkavy, and Lawrence, a law firm in Raleigh with attorneys who handled civil rights cases. One of the paralegals, Alyssa Gsell, was willing to listen to my story, and after several follow-up questions, she asked me to meet with a lawyer named

Burton Craige. All three of us sat down about a week before I left North Carolina, and the two of them asked me still more questions about what had happened before, during, and after I was a student at UNC. It took another month and more queries on their part before Burton decided to take my case on contingency.

In the meantime, I pursued my complaint with OCR. Two people from the agency contacted me and asked for more details about what happened as my documents worked their way through the system. I was encouraged that OCR was taking my situation seriously, but the staffers who followed up with me did not seem to have experience in handling complaints about hearing loss issues. One of the OCR employees had a son with a learning disability, and the other did not indicate that he had any background in accommodations for students who are Deaf or hard of hearing. They meant well, and I appreciated their time. But I was not optimistic that OCR would be able to resolve the issues that I had with UNC.

It was gratifying and heartwarming nonetheless that many people, including several of my former professors, wrote letters of support on my behalf to OCR. U.S. Senators Dianne Feinstein (D-CA) and Jesse Helms (R-NC) wrote to OCR to follow up on my complaint against UNC, and Tom Harkin (D-IA) gave written support to my persisting in challenging UNC's noncompliance with federal disability law as well. Brenda Battat, then deputy executive director of Self Help for Hard of Hearing People Inc. (later the Hearing Loss Association of America) wrote in a December 22, 1997, letter to OCR:

> UNC was totally unresponsive to Ms. Laufer's needs as a student with a hearing loss and ignored her rights as provided for by Federal laws . . . All of the requests that Ms. Laufer made of UNC are within her legislative rights . . . SHHH supports Ms. Laufer's claim. From the facts presented to us and as we understand them we believe that she was discriminated against and that UNC should be held accountable. SHHH understands very well the frustrations Ms. Laufer has gone through unnecessarily. We urge you to move ahead with

resolving her complaint as quickly as possible. (Brenda Battat, Self Help for Hard of Hearing People, letter to the U.S. Department of Education, Office for Civil Rights, December 22, 1997)

While OCR was processing my complaint, Burton Craige was preparing a civil action to file in the United States District Court, for the Middle District of North Carolina. We filed the lawsuit on March 18, 1998, naming the Board of Governors of the University of North Carolina as the defendant and alleging "discrimination on the basis of disability under the Rehabilitation Act of 1973 . . . and Title II of the Americans with Disabilities Act."[4] Because the substance of my OCR complaint and my civil lawsuit were the same, OCR ceased action on my complaint. I was hoping that my lawsuit would prevent anyone else from having to go through the discrimination I experienced, even though I knew that litigation would likely be a long and painful process.

And it was. For the next seven months my life was consumed by discovery requests, interrogatory responses, faxes, and depositions. If you think that litigation is the lights-camera-action glamour that those afternoon judge shows portray, think again. Lawsuits are neither fun nor exciting, especially when your civil rights are at stake. They are excruciating and arduous. I was up until three and four in the morning on countless nights responding to interrogatories sent to me by the North Carolina associate attorney general who was representing UNC.

This same attorney deposed me for fourteen hours over two days, asking a notebook full of questions covering just about every minute that I was in Chapel Hill, as well as a lot of my time before and after my withdrawal from UNC. The transcript of my deposition was 435 pages long. I do not think I have ever been so tired as I was at the end of that second day of my testimony. I was required to disclose almost every facet of my life, ranging from my academic records to my medical information, salary, hearing dog's veterinary file, and personal e-mails between my friends and me.

The more the associate attorney general probed, the stronger my case became. The more Burton investigated, the stronger my case became. Everything that I had said was consistent with my documentation and what others told the lawyers, with the exception of UNC maintaining that I had never requested specific accommodations and that they had no record of such a request from me.

But the day came when Burton deposed UNC's vice chancellor for student services—the one with whom I had met several weeks before I withdrew from the university, and the person I had seen actually write down a list of what I needed to hear in my courses. She had written the list on the back of a letter that I had sent; she apparently used that sheet to make notes during our meeting. UNC produced the letter in one of Burton's discovery requests. When Burton showed the vice chancellor the list, she did not deny that it was her writing, and I felt vindicated at last.

We were in mediation the next day (the mediation was required as a way to avoid a trial, and our mediation date had been pre-scheduled). I was adamant about not settling merely for money. I wanted to be reimbursed for what I had paid UNC in tuition and fees—as well as moving expenses and related costs associated with my time in Chapel Hill—but it was equally important for me to make it harder for UNC to treat any other student the same way.

After several hours of negotiating, UNC's attorneys agreed to create a steering committee comprised of university professors and officials. The committee was responsible for hiring at least one consultant to conduct a review of the Chapel Hill campus with respect to UNC's compliance with the Americans with Disabilities Act and the Rehabilitation Act. The review was to evaluate compliance matters germane to all students, not just students with hearing loss. The consultant or consultants were also required to issue a public report about the review, including nonbinding recommendations, by July 1, 1999.

The consultant's report identified many problems, including issues with documentation procedures, program accessibility, and adaptive technology. With respect to the accommodations provided in graduate and professional programs, the consultant found that, "There are no consistent policies or practices identified regarding the provision of notice to students, referral of students for services or the actual delivery of services. The present process of serving students with disabilities leaves the University extremely vulnerable to legal challenges."[5]

UNC offered me $100,000 as the other part of my settlement, though it did not admit liability. After legal fees—of which Burton earned every penny—and totaling up what the experience had cost me from start to finish, I pretty much broke even on the financial side. But we settled the lawsuit less than a year after we filed it—a much shorter length of time than I was expecting for resolution at the beginning—and getting that consultant's review was a victory in my mind and in my heart.

As I read the consultant's report, it dawned on me that I had told several people at UNC many of the same things not quite two years earlier, and for free. Whether or not UNC modified its policies and processes after the report was issued is a question only people on the Chapel Hill campus can answer. I have not been back there—it is still very painful to remember what happened to me—but I hope that they learned a big nonacademic lesson and that students with disabilities can flourish on that campus. These students deserve no less.

Remote-Controlled Professors

As a happy footnote to what happened at UNC, I want to share the funny side of attending college with a hearing loss. Here are my most memorable moments:

Professor W was eight months pregnant on the first day of the semester. With each class meeting before she gave birth, my ALD clip became harder and harder for the professor to attach to her maternity clothing. When she forgot to give my ALD back after class about three weeks into the term, I started after her as she walked back to her office. She was moving pretty slowly by that time, so it didn't take me much time at all to catch up to her. She was a great sport about everything!

Professor X used to put my ALD battery pack in the front pocket of his pants, in which he also kept his keys. He had a nervous habit of jangling the keys during his lectures, which inevitably caused him to accidentally hit the "off" switch on the ALD right in the middle of a sentence about essential material that was sure to crop up on the next exam or problem set. My friend Kai and I worked out a hand-waving signal for the professor for whenever the ALD went off; I would wave like a Rose Parade Queen to get the professor's attention, and Kai, bless him, would take copious notes during the "off" time so that I wouldn't miss any material.

Professor Y adored Chelsey, my first hearing dog. At the end of lecture one day, the professor asked the class if anyone had any questions. No one said anything, and we still had a couple of minutes left before the class period ended (yes, he *would not* let us go early). After a long pause, our instructor turned to Chels and asked her if *she* had any questions. Chelsey perked right up and bayed in her finest Siberian husky voice, "ArrroUUUUgggh-hhhh." Two hundred students roared so loudly that I could feel the guffaws in my seat.

Professor Z almost murdered me. I destroyed his planned grand exit on the last day of lecture. He had a whole speech prepared, which he delivered with aplomb and panache—think of the words in Dr. Seuss's *Oh, The Places You'll Go!* with a Henry Higgins-esque attitude—and he ended his monologue with a deep, heartfelt, "Farewell, all." He bowed, and walked slowly to the door as we all applauded. I thought he was going to stop, I swear, but he kept on going, with my ALD microphone still attached as he headed off to Hawaii or who knows where for the long winter break.

I shouted after him, "Professor! You have my microphone! I need it for my next class!"

He paused, still with his back to everyone, and I could see his shoulders droop in disappointment; the actor/bard in him was clearly peeved at my rude interruption of his performance. How do I know for sure? Because as he turned around and unclipped my ALD, he said through gritted teeth, "Sara, thank you for ruining my adieu."

I saw my grade point average swirling down the drain.

9

Relationships: The Ecstasy Without the Agony

HAVING A HEARING loss can present relationship challenges that require sensitivity and thoughtful communication skills. If you are already in a relationship and a hearing loss manifests itself in one or both partners, the changes that both people experience can be stressful and saddening at times. Above all else, a hearing loss is indeed a loss. Grieving and mourning your loss are

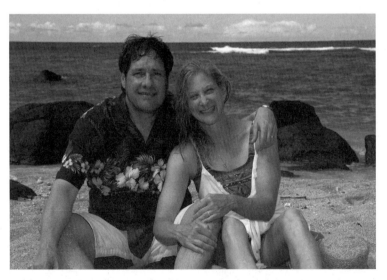

The author and her husband, John, during their honeymoon on Kauai. Yes, you can wear a hearing aid at the beach! Just take it off and put it in a zip-top bag before you go into the water. Photo credit: © 2008 John S. Batinovich. All rights reserved.

normal. You no longer have something that you used to have, and that something has been very important to your identity and to your connection to the world. Adjusting to the loss takes time and patience. It is natural to miss your hearing and all that it provided.

Casual interactions, whether talking to the produce manager at your local supermarket or saying hello to a neighbor across the street, also will be different after you notice a problem with your hearing. While these more ephemeral moments are less significant than the communications with your family and significant others, they are still difficult when your hearing loss alters their momentum—asking people to repeat themselves, misunderstanding directions, and not hearing more than bits and pieces can be annoying to others and confusing for everybody.

This chapter offers ways for improving communication in your relationships and contains several tips for smoothing the bumps in the conversation highways that you travel each day.

What to Do When Other People Deny Your Hearing Loss

People close to you will miss your hearing almost as much as you do, and they will be going through many of the same frustrations. Sometimes it is easy for a spouse, partner, or friend to make assumptions about what a person with a hearing loss can still hear—some of that is wishful thinking—and altering those expectations and their subsequent behaviors is not easy.

People you have known for a long time and who remember you from when your hearing was better may not understand or accept that you have trouble hearing, especially if you can still speak clearly. They may have unrealistic expectations, such as wanting you to have long (or any) phone conversations or to hang out in sports bars like the two of you did years before.

Acknowledge the other's confusion—it is valid and understandable—and assure her or him that your hearing loss is a barrier to communication, but it does not change your feelings about the person or the relationship that the two of you have developed over such a long time. Clearly explain your needs and limits, describe how you can best communicate, and discuss what the other person can do to help. Here are a few suggestions:

- Ask others to face you so that you can speechread. It is usually more effective when people speak slower rather than louder. Ask with a smile, not with an exasperated expression on your face.
- Converse away from background noise as much as possible, including other people's conversations as well as traffic, restaurant, and other ambient noise. Many of today's hearing aids are able to suppress background noise, but they are also designed to isolate and amplify the human voice. If you are trying to hear one person in the midst of many, your hearing aid won't know which one you need to listen to, so it will be hard to distinguish one particular speaker.
- Suggest to those in your inner circle that they call out your name before saying something so that you are "alerted" to their forthcoming words.
- Remember that sound dissipates rapidly with increasing distance, so try to be no more than a few feet from whomever is speaking unless you are using an assistive listening device.
- Educate everyone at home about assistive devices that you are using, or soon will be, such as lamp flashers to let you know when someone is at the door or a phone amplifier (if you share a phone, remember to turn down the volume when you end a call!). If you use an FM or infrared system at home, show your family members how to use the microphone. Keep all small parts and batteries away from children and pets.
- Let your friends and family members know that you need to keep phone calls short (or if you are having too much difficulty hearing to use the phone at all) and suggest e-mails or good old-fashioned letters as alternatives.
- Offer to pick restaurants that are quieter, and make the reservation yourself; request a table away from the kitchen and other high-traffic areas. Sitting outdoors, weather permitting, can be lovely.

- Give yourself time to get used to how your own voice sounds with your amplification when you get hearing aids or a cochlear implant. It may seem that your voice is quite loud in some situations and barely a whisper in others. Your friends and relatives can let you know when you need to modulate your speech in different environments.
- Rely on your training agency for guidance about integrating a canine companion into your home routine if you get a hearing dog. Most agencies will interview everyone in your household prior to placing a service dog with you and give everyone an opportunity to ask questions.

You do not need to apologize for your listening limitations, nor should you. Some people, regardless of how long you have known them, can—frankly—be insensitive about your situation, and they will not appreciate that you can converse more easily in person or without background noise than you can on the phone or in a noisy restaurant. If you sense that someone is in denial about your hearing loss, and if explaining your situation does not help, you may need to establish and maintain a boundary rather than try to be a martyr by enduring situations that are not working or healthy for you. You can't change anyone except yourself, and to try to do so will be a destructive and self-destructive effort. Back off for a while and nurture your other relationships. Reach out again after some time passes, if you feel comfortable trying to rebuild the friendship.

Practicing Proactivity in Your Daily Life

Many times in past years I did not want to participate in a social activity or go to an event because of my hearing loss, and because of how much background noise and insensitive people bothered me. I have worried about everything from whether or not I'll be able to hear anyone to what people will think when they see someone younger with hearing aids or a cochlear implant (and people do stare, everywhere). I turned down lots of invitations and missed a lot of opportunities because of these fears before the longing of not being with my friends or relatives got to be too much, and I finally reached a point where I had to try to make a change for the better.

The philosopher Aristotle was a master of classifying and categorizing, and after I took a rhetoric class where his *Rhetoric* was required reading—yes, the whole book—I got the idea to try to deal with my reluctance to have a social life by penciling out a more structured way of managing my feelings. I sorted out what was going on, why it was a problem, what I could do about it, and what happened after I tried to do something—anything—to get involved in an activity. Putting everything down on paper pulls the negative feelings out of me, and seeing them in front of me neutralizes them in a way; they aren't as bad in words on a notepad as they are in my head!

My solutions haven't always worked, but doing something *and* doing nothing are both choices that I have, and usually, the former is the better option for me. (I am not very good at doing nothing.) Writing down what happened after I try a possible solution gives me a record of my accomplishments, however minor they have often been, and that is an empowering feeling. When I am faced with a similar challenge or fear that I've dealt with before, I refer back to my notes and take the plunge to enjoy new experiences. And when I come up against a new obstacle, I have more confidence that I can work through it.

The following table may help you, too. Try not to be absolute in your thinking and writing—flexibility is important. Aristotle also wrote, in the *Nicomachean Ethics*, that "the rule adapts itself to the shape of the stone and is not rigid."[1] Those are wise words to keep in mind when something that you try doesn't work as you planned that it would.

Think about a situation in which listening was difficult for you, and when you chose not to participate. In the worksheet in figure 20, describe the situation and your concerns in the first column. List specific obstacles in the second column and possible solutions in the third—brainstorm here, and don't worry about your ideas

Situation	Specific Obstacles	Possible Solutions	Outcome
My family and I are going to an amusement park in a couple of weeks, and I am worried that my hearing aids will fall off if I go on the roller coasters.	1. My hearing aids may fly off of my ears.	1. I can put my hearing aids in their case, and put the case in a zip-top plastic bag in my fanny pack.	I was nervous about asking the ride operator for special assistance, but I told her about my hearing loss, and she was really nice and helpful. She even offered to hold onto my hearing aid case while all of us went on the coaster.
What if my aids get lost? And what if other people there make fun of me? Maybe I shouldn't even go!	2. I won't be able to hear safety instructions.	2. I can ask one of the ride operators ahead of time for instructions.	It was fun! I don't even know if anyone was staring at me.
	3. People may laugh at me, or point at my ears.	3. My family will be right there, and we can ignore any rude people.	
	1	1	
	2	2	
	3	3	
	4	4	
	5	5	

Figure 20. Practicing proactivity—a consciousness-raising activity.

seeming silly or unrealistic. If you can conceive of it, you can often make it happen. See the first part for an example.

The next time the opportunity to participate in that event or occasion happens, try one or more of your possible solutions and see what happens. Write the outcome down in the fourth column and assess how you feel. Even if things didn't work out perfectly, were you glad that you gave it a shot? Perfection isn't the goal—consciousness raising and confidence building are more important to develop a sense of control over your feelings and authority over your actions.

What to Do If Someone Close to You Has an Untreated Hearing Loss, or Is Being Stubborn about Wearing Hearing Aids

Someone close to me, whom I have known for decades—I'll call her "Mom," to keep things anonymous—has an age-induced hearing loss, and she has two digital hearing aids. Mom has a habit of keeping her hearing aids in her purse instead of her ears, because she does not like to wear the devices when she does not think that she needs to hear (her offspring, etc.). Mom's purse can hear really, really well, but Mom struggles, and it can drive me a little crazy sometimes. I think that her behavior may be payback for my teenage years, but I am not sure.

What do you do in such a situation, besides biting your tongue and gritting your teeth in exasperation? Try these ideas:

- Sit down with the person and express your concern for his or her well-being. There are safety issues that you can bring up, such as the person not being able to hear a siren or cars honking in traffic.
- Try to find out the source of reluctance. Is it stigma, embarrassment, or cost concerns (if someone does not yet have hearing aids), or is there a problem with the hearing aids that can be fixed? Feedback is the source of incredible annoyance among people who wear hearing aids, and sometimes it can get so bad that not wearing the aids is preferable. Feedback can be

caused by something as simple as a piece of tubing in the earmold that has cracked with normal wear, an issue that takes just a few minutes to resolve. Other minor problems include not realizing that the batteries have died, wax buildup on the hearing aids, and difficulty using the telecoil setting in order to use the phone. A quick trip to the hearing aid dispenser can clear up these matters on the spot.

- Offer to help with listening practice. You can call your friend on the phone, for instance, and let him listen to your recognizable voice. Tell a favorite story or say something else that is recognizable so that there is context for the words in the absence of speechreading.

- Accompany a loved one to the audiologist. Let him or her know that support is available and that he or she is not alone. Hearing loss is very isolating and maintaining a network can make a world of difference in how successful someone becomes in managing day-to-day challenges. Going to the audiologist together will also give you a chance to ask questions that you may have about your role in your companion's listening rehabilitation or about the hearing aid or cochlear implant technology.

- Check into alternatives and supplements to hearing aids, such as television amplification headphones, amplified telephones, vibrotactile alarm clocks, and visual alerting devices. These pieces of equipment can help in specific situations, and they are better than nothing if someone flat-out refuses to wear hearing aids.

- If your loved one lives alone, let his or her neighbors know about the hearing loss. Give them your phone number or e-mail address in case of an emergency.

- Ask someone you know who wears hearing aids or a cochlear implant to spend some time with your family member, so that he or she can appreciate the benefit that the devices can make in everyday life.

- Watch for any other symptoms of illness since the effects of stress—as seen in chapter 4—are profound. Pay attention to how your relative is coping and encourage prompt medical attention if either of you notices any new symptoms of illness. Find out if there is a support group for people with hearing loss at your loved one's health care provider; if not, suggest starting one.

- Take advantage of help from advocacy organizations and community support groups, such as the Hearing Loss Association of America (HLAA) and the Association of Late-Deafened Adults (ALDA). Local chapters across the country have regular meetings, and both you and your friend or relative can get a lot of good information and resources by talking to members. See the links to HLAA and ALDA in appendix B.

Romance with a Hearing Loss

If you have a hearing loss and enter into a new relationship, from the first meeting you will need to make your listening needs known and be patient as the relationship develops in ways that are likely new to both of you. Preconceived beliefs that both of you may have can turn out to be unfounded or far more minor than either of you expected.

You may, for example, think that a new beau will be unwilling to speak slowly or to face you consistently so that you can speechread, and that she or he may question whether or not you will be able to do typical "date" activities like dancing and going to concerts. Being willing to talk through your needs and to respond with consideration to another's needs will go a long way toward building a solid foundation for a happy and healthy relationship.

Sometimes, though, a person will not be comfortable continuing a relationship with a person with a hearing loss. Those breakups are excruciating. In such a circumstance, it is important (though perhaps not very comforting) to know that the breakup is not your fault and that you will be better off moving on to a relationship where you can be loved and appreciated for who you are, ears and all. There is no perfect person, and all of us have issues and problems that we can either choose to face and manage, or to deny and ignore.

Working through obstacles as an individual and as a couple takes a lot of work, but the results sure are worth it. Following are several tips to enrich your relationships with loving and sensitive communication.

- Do your part to make conversation as enjoyable as possible. Put fresh batteries in your devices before an important talk or date.
- Know when you communicate best. If you are not a morning person, try to have longer talks in the afternoon or evening.
- Plan activities that are fun but that take place in quieter surroundings. Picnics, game nights, and hikes make for fun dates that are easy on your ears.
- Don't avoid events you want to attend. If you want to go dancing or to a concert, you can still have a great time! If the music is too loud, take out or turn off your hearing aids or speech processor and appreciate the events using your other senses.
- Use your sense of touch and your sense of humor to create your own nonverbal language with your partner for the times when you are not wearing your hearing aids or cochlear implant, such as when you are in bed or in the shower. Decide on tactile signals for emergencies, too. By working together to find solutions that work for both of you, you and your partner can both bridge the hearing gap and become closer as a couple.
- Can your hearing aids pass the "hug test"? If you get feedback when you hug someone, you may need new earmold impressions, earmold tubing, or hearing aid reprogramming. Make an appointment with your audiologist before Valentine's Day!
- Tackle home modifications as a team. Rearrange your living room furniture so that the sun doesn't shine in your face and make speechreading difficult, consider carpeting to absorb background noise, and add visual alerts such as strobelight smoke alarms.
- Going through a rough patch because of listening troubles? Make an extra effort to do something special for yourself. Keep a list of simple pleasures that make you feel good and that don't require hearing—such as meditating, reading a favorite poem, or sipping iced tea outside—and do one every day.

- If stresses or events get to be too much to handle on your own, seek professional help. There is no shame in working through your troubles with a counselor or a therapist, and potentially a lot of good can come from this life-management strategy.

A Tale of Romance with a Hearing Loss

My husband and I met through an online dating service. I was the last person who expected to find the love of my life this way, and I mean the rock-bottom, sludge in the sewer, dregs in the coffee pot *last* person. I am far from an expert on matters pertaining to Cupid, having made more stupid mistakes in the name of love over the years than I care to remember—but that I can't seem to forget—and I had major doubts that I would meet my soul mate electronically.

I signed up with an online service grudgingly, and then only because my Auntie Nancy and my primary care doctor, of all people, egged me on. But to paraphrase John Lennon, life happens when you make plans, and the cyberspace path to love worked out well for me. (And yes, Auntie Nancy and the good doctor are patting themselves on the back.)

I did, however, have to kiss a few frogs along the way, and I met a few others who did not want to date a woman with a hearing loss. My philosophical attitude now, with the perspective of 20/20 hindsight, is that it was their loss. At the time, though, it was very painful to be rejected simply because of my hearing, although I knew not to settle for less than I deserved, just because of my ears.

When I took the plunge into the online dating pool, I was cautious. I did not include that I have a hearing loss in my dating profile. Most of the time when I would start communicating with a guy, I brought up my hearing aids early in the process. A couple of times, I never heard back, and one immature joker responded, "CAN YOU HEAR ME IF I TYPE IN ALL CAPITAL LETTERS?" which ended that string of e-mails. After that, I stopped mentioning my ear issues until I met a guy in person, at which point the topic was unavoidable. (Read more about that in "The Jimi Hendrix Effect" at the end of this chapter.)

My e-mails with John (my aforementioned most excellent husband) were different from the beginning. His first question to me was, "What kinds of music do you like?" After cringing and grimacing at my computer terminal and hemming and hawing for a few minutes and pigging out on ice cream, I decided to tell John about my ears, my hearing dog, and even my vibrotactile alarm clock and the strobe light smoke alarms at home. I fully expected to never to hear back from him—on top of living in a different state, he was (and still is) a huge rock and roll fan—but son of a gun, he responded a few hours later and made no issue of my ears. John liked dogs, and he e-mailed me photos of his beloved cat, Sam.

In cyberdating, of course, the written word is primary, and I didn't know how things would work out when John and I started to talk on the phone, and when we met in person several weeks later. The phone is tough for me, but I had prepped John about speaking slowly, and fortunately, I could comprehend his deep voice long-distance, with some "whats?" from me punctuating our talk. We conversed at first about subjects about which we had e-mailed, so having that familiarity also helped me to piece together information that my ears missed on the phone.

We have had several challenges, from my not hearing John from a few inches away while at a noisy football stadium—he still does not know how I could not hear him shouting my name, and I still do not know how he expected me to pick out his voice from 70,000 screaming others—to having day-to-day conversations from more than a few feet away. Sometimes, I need to remind him that I am clinically deaf, and once in a while, my ears can indeed try John's patience. (I remind him that I am "going offline" when I take off my hearing aid and cochlear implant speech processor, and he keeps the Jeff Beck CDs turned down when we are both in his car!) By concentrating on our strengths, though, and by recognizing that all relationships have problems and challenges, we have made my hearing loss and John's passion for rock and roll mesh pretty well. He can dance way better than I can, but I can rock out without a care in the world about how wacky I look on the dance floor!

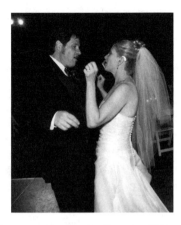

The author—dancing as only a hard of hearing White girl can!—with her husband on their wedding day; note the author's hearing aid. Photo credit: © 2008 Joe Buissink. All rights reserved.

The Jimi Hendrix Effect

Just about everyone who wears hearing aids has experienced the "Jimi Hendrix Effect." And it has nothing to do with music, in stark contrast to Jimi's all-too-brief contributions to the world. Engage in a meaningful hug with someone and revel in the high-pitched, pulsating "EeeahhrjjjhoooEEEEEzhzhzhzhzhzEEEEE" in the hugged ear. Pull a hat down a little too low and get the same thrill in stereo. Do something really inspired like take your hearing aids out of your ears before turning them off, and be rewarded by an electronic riff playing right from the palms of your hands that would make Jimi proud. Now try doing one or more of the above on a date, and you may see your social life evaporate.

My dating days are over, but the Jimi Hendrix Effect was a perennial concern of mine during those early stages of John's and my relationship, and for years before that. (Now, Jimi is only an occasional nuisance; his legend lives on, but it doesn't stress me out as much.) I had a lot of adventures with online dating before John's picture popped up on my screen.

One of my favorites was when my online dating service friend Keith and I got to the two-week mark of our virtual fact-finding mission, and Keith broached the subject that I both welcomed and dreaded: the first call.

"Soooooo," he wrote, with all of those o's illuminating his nervousness, "What do you think about talking on the phone?" I waited a few hours before responding. I was apprehensive too. Keith did not know about my ears yet, and I was not sure when or if to tell him before we met. Hearing aids can be the world's greatest dude repellant—not always a bad thing, like having a family full of lawyers—juxtaposed against my ability to make homemade chocolate truffles, a skill that is often a dude magnet. It's a push. Virtual dating wipes out the need for speechreading, and the problem of background noise, and all of the other annoying communications obstacles that I encounter whenever I talk with someone in person. But virtual dates don't hug back, and they don't kiss worth a damn, either.

At some point I would have to meet Keith with all five of my senses and see/hear/etc. how things went, or I would have to write him off having known him only one-dimensionally. Curiosity was a big incentive. I couldn't help but wonder if he really was all that he said he was—never married, doing social work that he absolutely loves, and into books and baseball and dogs and political activism and chocolate—or if his life was as superficial as his online picture, which looked like it was pilfered from a photo frame at Target.

I finally wrote back, "Cool. But I don't give out my phone number, I only exchange it. So you send me yours and I'll send you mine." At least I'd have the digits to give to my online dating SOS network in case Keith turned out to be featured on the post office bulletin board instead of a retail shelf. He agreed, so we swapped cell phone numbers and arranged for that first call; he would ring at 8:00 the next evening. I rested my ears most of that day, put in fresh phone amplifier batteries, and cranked up the phone handset volume as high as it would go. Necessary coping strategies to be sure, though I felt a little like I was perpetuating the myth of having normal hearing. I rationalized by telling myself that Keith had probably been telling me a few stretched truths himself. What a marvelous foundation for dating.

And with that wonderfully positive, barely cynical attitude, I waited for the phone to ring. And yes, I had put on makeup for the occasion; a phone date is still a date. Two minutes before 8:00, I dropped a dog treat by the phone table so that my hearing service dog, Bogie, would be ready to go to work when the phone rang. He is usually terrific about bounding to the phone without having a treat waiting as bait, but I wanted to preempt any potential snafus for this all-important first call. The phone rang at 8:03 according to the clock on the microwave, and Bogie, well-aware of the goodie with his name on it, zoomed over to the phone, barreled back to me and bonked my knee urgently with his strong snout, and then raced back to the ringer. I gave him another treat and thanked him before picking up the receiver and switching on my hearing aid telecoil.

"EEEEReeeeoooazhzhjjjhooo," the e-Jimi screeched—oh, *good grief shut up shut up shut up*, I pled silently; Jimi just had to have the first word. And I had to acknowledge his unavoidable presence by rolling the phone receiver around my ear until Jimi found that sweet spot where he and my hearing aid were at peace. I was grateful that he clammed up before I said hello to Keith. Maintain the fiction. After that, the conversation was in comparison boring, predictable, innocuous, and almost anticlimactic (it's nice to finally sort of meet you, how was your day, yes, the traffic was awful coming home, etc., etc.). Keith's voice was—as accurately as a medically deaf person can assess, anyway—friendly and engaging and just interesting enough to nudge me to meet him in person and find out if his voice matched everything else. And Keith sounded a whole lot less irritating than the synthetic Jimi, no offense to the legend.

We met for coffee the next Saturday afternoon. I still hadn't told Keith about my hearing aids by the time I got to the cafe, having decided to take my chances that my bionic ears wouldn't matter to him. Keith didn't know about Bogie either, even though the latter had made it clear with his almost parental eyes that he wanted to meet my virtual friend and assess whether or not he was worthy of us. Bogie knows what it means when I wear makeup for a telephone call. But I left him at home to watch cartoons for this first—and perhaps only—date, to avoid overwhelming a guy who had seemed decent so far.

The Target picture turned out to be pretty close to the real deal. Keith had a little less hair, and more of what was left was gray, but his face had character and depth, which I liked—and he was otherwise as advertised. I wasn't, as Jimi announced with an almost maniacal glee as Keith and I spotted each other in the coffeehouse and hugged lightly. As my ear brushed against Keith's cheek, Jimi introduced himself with a scene stealing, "RRRRRraaaaaaahzghgzghzeee," prompting me to pull back with an embarrassed shrug.

"It's just my hearing aids," I said, expecting Keith to run. "They have this feedback sometimes when they press up against anything." Keith was silent. I was scoring major points, ten seconds into our date. That's a new record for me. I tried to fill the awkwardness. "I call it the Jimi Hendrix Effect," I said with a patently manufactured smile. Still nothing. I decided to lay all of my cards on the table, since it looked like my hand was close to folding anyway. "I started to lose my hearing when I was a teenager, but I do pretty well with my hearing aids," I told him. "And I also want to tell you that I have a hearing service dog, but I left him at home for our date."

Ah, that triggered something. Keith's eyebrows rose all the way to his receding hairline. Good old Bogie was going to save the day, maybe. "You have a *what* dog?" he asked.

"A hearing service dog," I repeated. "He is trained to alert me to the phone and the doorbell and other sounds. He let me know the phone was ringing when you called the other night."

"Ahhhhh," he said, giving me that vacant stare that I've seen a million times, the one people use when their minds are processing the concept of a hearing dog. (She's not blind. What does she need a guide dog for?) "Does he screech too?" he finally asked.

That made me laugh, and Keith smiled too. "Only when he doesn't like the guy I'm with," I told him with a wink. "You'd better treat me right, or he'll know when I get home." The wink did it. We sat down for coffee in a quiet area of the cafe and had a nice chat. I still didn't know if his name really was Keith, but I decided to give things a chance and find out more about him.

We dated for a few months before Keith (not his real name after all, but a girl's entitled to a few secrets and his name will remain one here) accepted a job out of state. He wasn't the love of my life—nor was I his—but we enjoyed our times together and wished one another well as our lives took us on different paths. When we hugged goodbye, Jimi gave one last, brilliant, brazen encore, and this time, Keith and I laughed.

Rock on, Jimi.

Conclusion: My Utopia

WILL INCREASED PROVISION of hearing aids and cochlear implants instantly reduce health care costs, improve social interaction, and raise the standard of living for people who are hard of hearing? No. Will greater access to affordable hearing health care improve overall health care and quality of life? Almost certainly. As I have shown, untreated hearing loss can have devastating physical, emotional, and social costs in the working ages.

These problems, if left underserved, will likely fester and become even bigger and more expensive when today's working-age population transitions into retirement. We need to deal with untreated hearing loss now. In particular, the hearing health care delivery system can be improved through labor and health provision enhancements. I touched briefly on my health care utopia in chapter 5, suggesting ways to improve health care delivery at the individual level. On the societal echelon, many more advancements are necessary to bring hearing health care into the 21st century. In my utopia, here is what will happen:

Well-documented is the importance of work to self-esteem. To increase labor force participation among people with hearing loss (and all disabilities), large businesses will establish "accessibility centers" in their human resource departments where people can try out phone amplifiers, large-print software at demonstration stations, ergonomic devices, and other commonly used accommodations by workers with all types of disabilities. When a hiring manager submits a requisition for a new desktop computer and office supplies, she or he will also requisition "work optimization equipment" for the new hire.

Removing the onus of having to request these small and inexpensive tools via a lengthy accommodations process will increase their use among new and existing workers, which will lead to reduced turnover, increased productivity, and higher employee morale. Smaller businesses will be served by government-funded accessibility centers located in urban centers and rural areas, or existing one-stop centers (federally funded career centers established by the Workforce Investment Act of 1998) with comprehensive assistive technology services on-site.

With respect to those of us who use (and the millions more who need) hearing aids and cochlear implants, if ear, nose, and throat doctors and audiologists maintain their heated rivalry for our business, we lose. Governing bodies and certifying organizations need to establish and enforce a distinct division of responsibilities belonging to each profession and make the segmentation clear to consumers. People with hearing loss need to know whom to see for specific conditions and care requirements. Government intervention in this process may be necessary because the professionals involved do not seem to be able to resolve the dispute over scope of practice matters by themselves.

Regulation of payment mechanisms may also be needed. If health insurance companies act on the evidence (see chapter 5) that hearing aid use may reduce expenditures for costly health conditions associated with hearing loss, such as depression, then they will offer benefits for hearing aids without delay. If they do not provide this coverage, then they may have to be forced to do so through government action that mandates third-party reimbursement. Shareholders in these companies should in the meantime question the reasoning capabilities of the firms' executives. Both federal and state governments have a strong incentive to implement a hearing health care mandate, because it may also reduce publicly funded health expenses among people in the working ages, and, in future decades, among the elderly. (If Medicare starts to cover hearing aids, present-day older adults may experience lower overall health care costs as well.)

As described in chapter 6, the military long ago showed how hearing health care improves the quality of life and vocational opportunities of veterans with hearing loss. The Department of

Veterans Affairs' (VA's) high-volume purchasing model is also cost-effective; as shown in chapter 3, the VA pays an average of $355 per hearing aid, while the average price of a hearing aid dispensed through retail channels is $1,676. Extrapolating this model to third-party payers makes sense, and it will probably save billions of dollars in both hearing health process improvements and in the costs of treating expensive comorbid conditions.

Dispensers can still charge whatever they want, but since cost is a barrier to getting hearing aids for about one-third of men and almost half of women under 67 years old (also shown in chapter 6), broad-based insurance coverage will drive more patients to get hearing aids by using health plan benefits. With adequate insurance benefits in place, dispensers can also enjoy substantial profits if they come up with ways to more efficiently serve patients.

Dispenser functions can be specialized so that efficiency improves. The usual practice is for one person to conduct hearing testing, make earmold impressions, perform minor repairs, describe different types of hearing aids and assistive listening devices, program hearing aids, instruct patients in how to use their aids, and offer help with speechreading, instead of having different employees specialize in these tasks, which require very different skills and knowledge.

Software engineers can develop products that will streamline the fitting process, and newly fitted patients can attend group classes or use online tutorials for guidance on the use and care of their hearing aids. Individual counseling will still be necessary, but not as often as is happening now, since most hearing aid and cochlear implant recipients are currently instructed one-on-one by dispensers and audiologists. Patients who want this custom service may have to pay out-of-pocket for it, and dispensers may be able to realize extra profits by offering "designer" services to customers willing to pay for them.

Manufacturers will also gain, because of the increased demand for their products and the potential for economies of scale on the production side. With existing policies, manufacturers have no reason to promote third-party coverage (although the Hearing

Industries Association, which is a trade association comprised of about thirty hearing device manufacturers,[1] supports the Hearing Aid Tax Credit),[2] because bigger profits are possible in the United States without it.

It is interesting to note the international penetration in U.S. hearing health care. Two of the three FDA-approved cochlear implant manufacturers are headquartered outside of the United States,[3] and about 40 percent of the hearing aid manufacturers listed on the Hearing Industries Association Web site are based in foreign countries.[4] All of these nations have universal health care systems, philosophically and administratively far different from health care in this country. From a pure business perspective, it is easy to see why manufacturers are not inclined to encourage federal involvement in hearing aid reimbursement policy here.

Hearing aid technology is proprietary, so a component designed for one brand of device will not work in products made by other manufacturers (the exceptions are disposable batteries, which come in standard sizes and can be used with any brand of hearing aid). That practice is not unusual—televisions, cell phones, and most appliances are made the same way—but when it comes time to repair a hearing aid, what a patient needs to do is time-consuming and inconvenient, because hearing aid manufacturers generally require that a dispenser send in a hearing aid needing repair. This effort takes time from a dispenser's day and necessitates extra trips by the consumer to the dispenser's office for this middleman service.

In my utopia, manufacturers will have retail locations for on-site repairs or satellite offices away from their headquarters to better serve customers. Consumers will communicate directly with the manufacturer when repairs are necessary, just like consumers do with almost every other product repair. Online, real-time customer service and troubleshooting assistance will be offered during normal business hours, and manufacturers will guarantee turnaround times for repairs.

As disabling as a hearing loss can be, it can also offer benefits. Compensatory sense development, compassion, creative problem solving, and resilience (not to mention chutzpah) are just a few attributes that people with hearing loss tend to develop as they live their lives. Burton Craige, the lawyer who represented me when I sued the University of North Carolina for disability discrimination, once passed along to me advice from one of his mentors: life is struggle. These words are true—however maddening it is at times to have a hearing loss, I also cannot think of anyone else I know or have ever met who is living a charmed existence. The trick is to thrive not merely in spite of a hearing loss—that has negative underpinnings that I can well do without—but because of a hearing loss.

Inertia is easy, and silence is easy to ignore. *Sound Sense* challenges the status quo, calling upon policy makers to increase access to hearing health care. This book also questions the merit of extant hearing health delivery practices and suggests more efficient and effective alternatives for patients and practitioners. Contradictions in practices hurt instead of help and are based upon avarice and ignorance in some cases, as opposed to evolving from enlightened solutions that can strengthen both individuals and society.

I hope that *Sound Sense* encourages, equips, and challenges working-age people with hearing loss to maximize ownership of their condition and their lives. No situation is perfect, but striving for improvement is always sublime.

How does that sound?

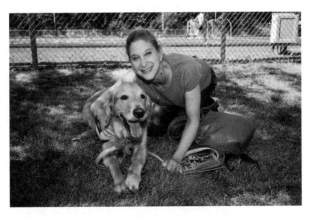

The author and her hearing dog, Bogie, taking a break after practicing their signal training. Photo credit: © 2009 John S. Batinovich. All rights reserved.

Appendix A

Technical Notes on Data Sources[*]

- Data for this book are from the 2007 and 2008 National Health Interview Survey (NHIS) Public Use Person and Sample Adult files, and were analyzed using Intercooled Stata v9.2 for the Macintosh.
- Data are self-reported by respondents or their proxies.
- Data sets were merged on the Household Serial Number (HHX), Family Number (FMX), and Person Number (FPX).
- The NHIS 2007 sample size for ages 18–66 is 19,397, and the sample size for all adults in the Sample Adult file is 23,393.
- The NHIS 2008 sample size for ages 18–66 is 17,932, and the sample size for all adults in the Sample Adult file is 21,781.
- The weight used for all analyses is the sample adult file final annual weight (WTFA_SA).
- Findings were not reported for unweighted cell counts less than 30.
- Unless otherwise noted, refused to answer, not ascertained, and don't know responses have been excluded from analyses.
- For more information on the NHIS, see http://www.cdc.gov/nchs/nhis.htm.

How the NHIS Collects Data from People Who Are Hard of Hearing

The NHIS follows a procedure for communicating with respondents who are Deaf or hard of hearing: "The NHIS is an in-person

---

[*] *Note*: In May 2010, the National Center for Health Statistics (NCHS) re-released the 2008 NHIS Sample Adult data file because of late corrections to final weight adjustments to fourth quarter data. NCHS has determined that annual estimates calculated from the re-released dataset do not result in noteworthy differences from those estimates calculated with the original dataset.

interview which stipulates that interviewers are supposed to make initial contact with the household in person. The sample is based on street addresses rather than phone numbers. There is some telephone follow-up allowed in the NHIS, however, if that is the preference of the respondent once initial contact has been made in person.

"While there is no specific policy for interviewers to follow when respondents have hearing or speech difficulties, they may adopt measures such as getting an interpreter or having the respondent sit next to them with the interview on the laptop in order to indicate answers to the questions."[1] (Centers for Disease Control and Prevention, National Center for Health Statistics, e-mail to the author, December 19, 2008)

Appendix B

Resources and Recommended Reading

Chapter 1: Listen While You Work

U.S. Equal Employment Opportunity Commission

Questions and Answers about Deafness and Hearing Impairments in the Workplace and the Americans with Disabilities Act, http://www.eeoc.gov/facts/deafness.html

Enforcement Guidance: Reasonable Accommodation and Undue Hardship Under the Americans with Disabilities Act, http://www.eeoc.gov/policy/docs/accommodation.html

U.S. Department of Justice

ADA Enforcement, http://www.ada.gov/enforce.htm

U.S. Department of Labor, Bureau of Labor Statistics

Occupational Outlook Handbook, 2010-11 Edition, http://www.bls.gov/OCO/

This Web page has links to overviews of hundreds of occupations, with information including the nuts and bolts of each job, working conditions, pay, and necessary training.

Occupational Outlook Handbook, 2010-11 Edition, State Sources http://www.bls.gov/oco/oco20024.htm

See this Web page for links to occupational and labor market information for each state and territory. Many state pages also have career exploration tools and links to resume submission pages for state jobs.

U.S. Department of Labor, Office of Disability Employment Policy

Job Accommodation Network, http://askjan.org/cgi-win/TypeQuery.exe?902

This Web site contains a listing of Vocational Rehabilitation (VR) departments by state, with links to the state VR websites.

U.S. Department of Veterans Affairs
Vocational Rehabilitation and Employment Service, http://www .vba.va.gov/bln/vre/

U.S. Small Business Administration, Office of Entrepreneurial Development, and U.S. Department of Justice, Civil Rights Division
ADA Guide for Small Businesses, http://www.ada.gov/smbustxt.htm

Writing Your Résumé
Susan Britton Whitcomb, *Résumé Magic: Trade Secrets of a Professional Resume Writer,* 4th ed. (St. Paul, Minn.: JIST Publishing, 2010).
Joyce Lain Kennedy, *Resumes for Dummies,* 5th ed. (Hoboken, NJ: Wiley Publishing, 2007).
These books offer expert advice on creating an effective résumé.

Chapter 2: Just Another Day in Auditory Paradise

Uploaded Videos: Adding/Editing Captions
YouTube Help, http://www.google.com/support/youtube/ bin/answer.py?answer=100077

National Center for Accessible Media
Media Access Generator (MAGpie), http://ncam.wgbh.org/ webaccess/magpie/

Online Directory—Find a State Equipment Program, http://www .tedpa.org/directory/?linkid=43
Telecommunications Equipment Distribution Program Association

Harris Communications, http://www.harriscomm.com/
Assistive devices and supplies for people who are Deaf or hard of hearing

Hearmore, http://www.hearmore.com/store/default.asp
Assistive devices and supplies for people who are Deaf or hard of hearing

Access to Movie Theaters for Patrons who are Deaf, Hard of Hearing, Blind or Visually Impaired, http://ncam.wgbh.org/mopix/nowshowing.html
MoPix Motion Picture Access/Media Access Group at WGBH
This Web site contains a directory of movie theaters in the U.S. equipped with Rear Window Captioning.

H.E.A.R., http://www.hearnet.com/index.shtml
Hearing Education and Awareness for Rockers

NPC Online Library, http://www.nonoise.org/library.htm
Noise Pollution Clearinghouse

Exemptions to the Closed Captioning Requirements on the Basis of Undue Burden, http://www.fcc.gov/cgb/dro/caption_exempt ions.html
Federal Communications Commission, Consumer and Governmental Affairs Bureau

Chapter 3: Getting a Hearing Aid or a Cochlear Implant, Demystified

Hearing Aids
U.S. Department of Health & Human Services, U.S. Food and Drug Administration, http://www.fda.gov/MedicalDevices/ProductsandMedicalProcedures/HomeHealthandConsumer/ConsumerProducts/HearingAids/default.htm
This new FDA Web site, designed especially for consumers, provides comprehensive information about hearing aids in easy-to-understand language, with links to additional resources.

Medical and Dental Expenses
Department of the Treasury, Internal Revenue Service Publication 502, http://www.irs.gov/publications/p502/
The IRS guide provides this guide for taxpayers, and it gives specific information on hearing health care expenses—such as hearing aids and hearing dog maintenance—that can be deducted from income taxes when tax filers meet the noted requirements.

Sound Advice on Hearing Aids
Federal Trade Commission, http://www.ftc.gov/bcp/edu/
pubs/consumer/health/hea10.shtm This site contains a helpful question and answer sheet on hearing aid purchasing.

Chapter 4: Sweat, Pump, Recharge, and Glow

Diane Ackerman, *A Natural History of the Senses,* (New York:
Vintage Books, 1995).
A wonderful book that shows how each of our senses has con-
tributed to past and present human existence.

Tempering Chocolate, http://www.ghirardelli.com/bake/choco
late_tempering.aspx
Tempering chocolate is a process of melting chocolate for coating
candies, so that the chocolate sets up looking shiny and clear
instead of dull and streaked. The instructions are on this Web site.

Chapter 5: To Your Health

Hearing Loss
U.S. National Library of Medicine and the National Institutes of
Health, MedlinePlus, http://www.nlm.nih.gov/medlineplus/
ency/article/003044.htm
This Web page gives a comprehensive list of medical causes of
hearing loss and an overview of what to anticipate at a doctor's appointment for a suspected hearing loss.

Chapter 6: When Silence Isn't Golden

The following journals are some of the leading audiology and
hearing aid trade publications. They offer interesting reading
on trends in hearing aid research, marketing, and politics.

Advance for Hearing Practice Management, http://audiology
.advanceweb.com

Ear and Hearing, http://journals.lww.com/ear-hearing/pages/
default.aspx

The Hearing Journal, http://www.audiologyonline.com/
theHearingJournal/

The Hearing Review, http://www.hearingreview.com

Chapter 7: Going to the Dogs

Martha Hoffman, *Lend Me an Ear: The Temperament, Selection, and Training of the Hearing Ear Dog* (Wilsonville, OR: Doral Publishing, 1999).
This book serves as a complete and helpful reference on hearing service dogs.

Washington State University College of Veterinary Medicine Pet Loss Support, http://www.vetmed.wsu.edu/PLHL/

Delta Society Pet Loss and Bereavement, http://www.deltasociety .org/Page.aspx?pid=307

Pet Loss Grief Support Website, http://www.petloss.com/

June Cotner, *Animal Blessings: Prayers and Poems Celebrating our Pets,* (New York: HarperCollins/HarperSanFrancisco, 2000).
For anyone who has lost a pet, this book will offer comfort and inspiration through words and a few photographs.

Chapter 8: Learning for a Lifetime

The Database of Accredited Postsecondary Institutions and Programs
U.S. Department of Education, Office of Postsecondary Education, http://ope.ed.gov/accreditation/Search.aspx

Tax Benefits for Education
Department of the Treasury, Internal Revenue Service Publication 970, http://www.irs.gov/publications/p970/
This publication from the IRS gives details on qualifying for tax credits for educational expenses.

Chapter 9: Relationships

Hearing Loss Association of America (HLAA), http://hearing loss.org.
HLAA advocates for better hearing health care policy, and it provides information to people with hearing loss on hearing

aids, assistive equipment, and coping strategies. Members can attend local chapter meetings nationwide.

Association of Late-Deafened Adults (ALDA), http://www.alda .org/
ALDA stresses flexible communication strategies for adults who are Deaf or severely hard of hearing. Local chapters are established throughout the United States.

Michael Harvey, *Listen with the Heart: Relationships and Hearing Loss,* (San Diego, CA: DawnSign Press, 2001).
Read this book for guidance on managing obstacles in personal relationships between people with and without hearing loss.

General Interest Reading on Hearing Loss and Disability

Susan Stoddard, Lita Jans, Joan M. Ripple, and Lewis Kraus, *Chartbook on Work and Disability in the United States, 1998,* (Washington, D.C: U.S. National Institute on Disability and Rehabilitation Research, 1998), http://www.infouse.com/ disabilitydata/workdisability/

Judith Holt, Sue Hotto, and Kevin Cole, *Demographic Aspects of Hearing Impairment: Questions and Answers,* 3rd ed., (Center for Assessment and Demographic Studies, Gallaudet University, 1994), http://research.gallaudet.edu/Demographics/ factsheet.php

Mary Lou Koelkebeck, Colleen Detjen, and Donald R. Calvert, *Historic Devices for Hearing: The CID-Goldstein Collection,* (St. Louis, MO: The Central Institute for the Deaf, 1984).
A thorough record of hearing aids and improvements to them over the years is offered in this book.

Marcia B. Dugan, *Living with Hearing Loss,* (Washington, DC: Gallaudet University Press, 2003).
Targeted toward older adults, this book is very well written and informative.

Notes

Introduction: A Silent Avalanche

1. Judy E. Yordon, *Roles in Interpretation*, 2nd ed. (Dubuque, IA: Wm C. Brown Publishers, 1989), 128–129.

2. B. S. Kisilevsky and others, "Fetal Sensitivity to Properties of Maternal Speech and Language," *Infant Behavior & Development* 32, no. 1 (2009): 59.

3. Integrated Public Use Microdata Series (IPUMS) USA, *The Census of 1850*, http://usa.ipums.org/usa/voliii/items1850.shtml (accessed July 20, 2010).

4. John Andrew Simpson and Edmund S. C. Weiner, *The Oxford English Dictionary*, 2nd ed., vol. 4 (1989; repr. with corrections, Oxford: Clarendon Press, 1998), 293–294.

5. Harlan Lane, *When the Mind Hears: A History of the Deaf* (New York: Vintage Books, 1989), 356–357.

6. Simpson and Weiner, *The Oxford English Dictionary*, vol. 1, 779–780.

7. Richard Butsch, *The Making of American Audiences: From Stage to Television, 1750–1990* (Cambridge: Cambridge University Press, 2000), 295.

8. Author analysis of 2007 National Health Interview Survey data. See appendix A for technical notes.

9. Author analysis of 2007 and 2008 National Health Interview Survey data. See appendix A for technical notes.

10. Author analysis of 2008 National Health Interview Survey data. See appendix A for technical notes.

11. Author analysis of 2008 National Health Interview Survey data (see appendix A for technical notes) and U.S. Census Bureau, "Detailed Data Files: Population Projections for 2000–2050," http://www.census.gov/population/www/projections/usinterimproj/usproj2000–2050.xls (accessed July 16, 2010).

12. Alice Walker, *Possessing the Secret of Joy* (New York: Pocket Books/Simon & Schuster, 1992), 281.

13. "Hear Well in a Noisy World: Hearing Aids, Hearing Protection & More," *Consumer Reports* 74, no. 7 (2009): 32.

14. Author analysis of 2008 National Health Interview Survey data. See appendix A for technical notes.

15. Author analysis of 2008 National Health Interview Survey data. See appendix A for technical notes.

16. Author analysis of 2007 National Health Interview Survey data. See appendix A for technical notes.

17. National Institutes of Health, National Institute on Deafness and Other Communication Disorders, "Long Description for New Cochlear Implants in 2001," April 3, 2008, http://www.nidcd.nih.gov/health/statistics/long-implants.htm (accessed September 10, 2009). Data are for ages 18–64 and include cochlear implant use for the Deaf and very hard of hearing persons. See documentation: National Institutes of Health, National Institute on Deafness and Other Communication Disorders, "New Cochlear Implants in 2001," http://www.nidcd.nih.gov/health/statistics/implants.htm (accessed September 10, 2009).

18. National Institutes of Health, National Institute on Deafness and Other Communication Disorders, "Cochlear Implants," August 31, 2009, http://www.nidcd.nih.gov/health/hearing/coch.htm#c (accessed September 10, 2009).

19. ASLInfo.com, "Deaf Time-Line: 1971–1988," http://www.aslinfo.com/trivia4.cfm (accessed February 26, 2009).

20. Kathleen E. Bainbridge, Howard J. Hoffman, and Catherine C. Cowle, "Diabetes and Hearing Impairment in the United States: Audiometric Evidence from the National Health and Nutrition Examination Survey, 1999–2004," *Annals of Internal Medicine* 149, no. 1 (2008): 1.

21. E. Tsakiropoulou and others, "Hearing Aids: Quality of Life and Socio-economic Aspects," *Hippokratia* 11, no. 4 (2007): 183.

22. Theresa Hnath Chisolm and others, "A Systematic Review of Health-Related Quality of Life and Hearing Aids: Final Report of the American Academy of Audiology Task Force on the Health-Related Quality of Life Benefits of Amplification in Adults," *Journal of the American Academy of Audiology* 18, no. 2 (2007): 151, 153.

23. David H. Kirkwood, "Economic Turmoil Threatens to Reverse Recent Growth in the Hearing Aid Market," *The Hearing Journal* 61, no. 12 (2008): 12.

24. "Hear Well in a Noisy World," *Consumer Reports*, 32–33.

25. Duke University Center for Demographic Studies, Medical Technology Assessment Working Group, *Assessing the Impact of Medical Technology Innovations on Human Capital: Phase I Final Report*

(Part G): Effects of Advanced Medical Technologies—Sensory Diseases, Hearing Impairment, Prepared for the Institute for Medical Technology Innovation, (January 2006): 4, 15.

26. George B. Haskell and others, "Subjective Measures of Hearing Aid Benefit in the NIDCD/VA Clinical Trial," *Ear and Hearing* 23, no. 4 (2002): 306.

27. Author analysis of 2007 National Health Interview Survey data. See appendix A for technical notes.

28. The British Society of Hearing Aid Audiologists (BSHAA), *Audiological Provision in Europe: A Public-Private Partnership?*, BSHAA Council, February 2005, http://www.hohadvocates.org/european report.pdf (accessed May 29, 2009), 4–5.

29. Medical News Today, "New NHS Focus On Audiology Brings Faster Hearing Aid Treatment," May 21, 2009, http://www.medical newstoday.com/articles/150979.php (accessed August 31, 2009).

30. Author analysis of 2007 National Health Interview Survey data. See appendix A for technical notes.

31. Kenneth C. Pugh, "Health Status Attributes of Older African-American Adults with Hearing Loss," *Journal of the National Medical Association* 96, no. 6 (2004): 777.

32. Carl Crandell, Terry L. Mills, and Ricardo Gauthier, "Knowledge, Behaviors, and Attitudes About Hearing Loss and Hearing Protection Among Racial/Ethnically Diverse Young Adults," *Journal of the National Medical Association* 96, no. 2 (2004): 176.

33. Author analysis of 2008 National Health Interview Survey data. See appendix A for technical notes.

34. Jed Boardman and others, "Work and Employment for People with Psychiatric Disabilities," *British Journal of Psychiatry* 182, no. 6 (2003): 467.

35. Social Security Administration, "Your Retirement Benefit: How It Is Figured," January 2010, *http://www.ssa.gov/pubs/10070.html* (accessed July 16, 2010).

36. Barbara Hoffmann and others, "Residential Traffic Exposure and Coronary Heart Disease: Results from the Heinz Nixdorf Recall Study," *Biomarkers* 14, no. S1 (2009): 74; Gösta Leon Bluhm and others, "Road Traffic Noise and Hypertension," *Occupational and Environmental Medicine* 64, no. 2 (2007): 122; Deepak Prasher, "Is There Evidence that Environmental Noise is Immunotoxic?," *Noise & Health* 11, no. 44 (2009): 153–154.

37. Author calculations of 2007 National Health Interview Survey data. See appendix A for technical notes.

38. Author calculations of 2007 National Health Interview Survey data. See appendix A for technical notes.

39. CBS News.com, "Hearing Loss Now A Military Epidemic," March 8, 2008, http://www.cbsnews.com/stories/2008/03/08/health/main3919311.shtml (accessed July 18, 2010).

40. Author calculations of 2008 National Health Interview Survey data. See appendix A for technical notes.

41. Author calculations of 2008 National Health Interview Survey data. See appendix A for technical notes.

42. Gary Robbins, "UCI finds way to ease severe ringing in the ears," *Orange County Register*, January 28, 2009.

43. National Institutes of Health, "Fact Sheet: Hair Cell Regeneration and Hearing Loss," September 2007, http://www.nih.gov/about/researchresultsforthepublic/Hair.pdf (accessed November 23, 2009).

44. Institute of Medicine of the National Academies, *100 Initial Priority Topics for Comparative Effectiveness Research*, 2009, http://www.iom.edu/~/media/Files/Report%20Files/2009/ComparativeEffectivenessResearchPriorities/Stand%20Alone%20List%200f%20100%20CER%20Priorities%20-%20for%20web.pdf (accessed July 18, 2010); World Health Organization, "WHO Calls on Private Sector to Provide Affordable Hearing Aids in Developing World," Press Release WHO/34, Jul. 11, 2001, http://who.int/inf-pr-2001/en/pr2001-34.html (accessed November 13, 2009).

45. Margaret I. Wallhagen and others, "An Increasing Prevalence of Hearing Impairment and Associated Risk Factors over Three Decades of the Alameda County Study," *American Journal of Public Health* 87, no. 3 (1997): 440.

Chapter 1: Listen While You Work

1. Nancy Tye-Murray, Jacqueline L. Spry, and Elizabeth Mauzé, "Professionals with Hearing Loss: Maintaining that Competitive Edge," *Ear and Hearing* 30, no. 4 (2009): 478.

Chapter 2: Just Another Day in Auditory Paradise

1. National Institutes of Health, National Institute on Deafness and Other Communication Disorders, *Noise: Keeping It Down at Home*, http://noisyplanet.nidcd.nih.gov/staticresources/materials/ParentTipsheet_KeepDownatHome.pdf (accessed November 2, 2009).

2. "Television: Larry Hagman: Vita Celebratio Est," *Time*, August 11, 1980, http://www.time.com/time/magazine/article/0,9171,924377,00.html (accessed November 2, 2009).

3. Author calculations of 2007 National Health Interview Survey data. Respondents had hearing that was neither excellent nor good, or hearing was good but worse in one ear than the other.

4. Federal Communications Commission, "Closed Caption Decoder Requirements for Analog Television Receivers," *Code of Federal Regulations*, Title 47, Vol. 1, sec. 15.119, revised October 1, 2005, 790–799, http://edocket.access.gpo.gov/cfr_2005/octqtr/47cfr15.119.htm (accessed November 2, 2009).

5. Federal Communications Commission, Consumer & Governmental Affairs Bureau, "Closed Captioning: FCC Consumer Advisory: Closed Captioning for Digital Television (DTV)," http://www.fcc.gov/cgb/consumerfacts/dtvcaptions.html (accessed July 14, 2010).

6. Federal Communications Commission, Consumer & Governmental Affairs Bureau, "Closed Captioning: FCC Consumer Facts," http://www.fcc.gov/cgb/consumerfacts/closedcaption.html (accessed November 2, 2009).

7. National Captioning Institute, e-mail message to author, August 4, 2009.

8. Author calculations of 2007 National Health Interview Survey data.

9. Author calculations of 2007 National Health Interview Survey data.

10. Dorothy Bruck and Ian R. Thomas, "Smoke Alarms for Sleeping Adults Who are Hard-of-Hearing: Comparison of Auditory, Visual, and Tactile Signals," *Ear and Hearing* 30, no. 1, (2009): 73.

11. U.S. Department of Transportation, Federal Aviation Administration, "Cochlear Implants Exempt from Rules Regarding 'Portable Electronic Devices,'" http://www.faa.gov/other_visit/aviation_industry/airline_operators/airline_safety/info/all_infos/media/2007/inF007022.pdf (accessed November 2, 2009).

Chapter 3: Getting a Hearing Aid or a Cochlear Implant, Demystified

1. U.S. Department of Health & Human Services, U.S. Food and Drug Administration, "Guidance for Industry and FDA Staff: Regulatory Requirements for Hearing Aid Devices and Personal Sound Amplification Products," February 25, 2009, http://www.fda.gov/MedicalDevices/DeviceRegulationandGuidance/GuidanceDocuments/ucm127086.htm (accessed November 20, 2009).

2. U.S. Department of Labor, Bureau of Labor Statistics, *Occupational Outlook Handbook, 2010–11 Edition,* http://www.bls.gov/oco/ocos085.htm (accessed July 19, 2010).

3. Audiology Online, "Federal Employee Hearing Aid Insurance Benefits Take Effect January 1," January 31, 2009, http://www.audiologyonline.com/news/news_detail.asp?news_id=3573 (accessed July 20, 2010).

4. American Speech-Language-Hearing Association, "State Insurance Mandates for Hearing Aids," http://www.asha.org/advocacy/state/issues/ha_reimbursement.htm (accessed July 17, 2010).

5. *The Patient Protection and Affordable Care Act,* Public Law 111–148, 111th Cong., 2d sess. (January 5, 2010), 45–46.

6. U. S. Department of Veterans Affairs, Denver Acquisition and Logistics Center, Veterans Health Information Systems and Technology Architecture data, e-mail message to author, June 20, 2009.

7. "Hear Well in a Noisy World: Hearing Aids, Hearing Protection & More," *Consumer Reports* 74, no. 7 (2009): 32–33.

8. U.S. Department of Veterans Affairs, Denver Acquisition and Logistics Center, Veterans Health Information Systems and Technology Architecture data, e-mail message to author, August 16, 2009.

9. U.S. Department of Veterans Affairs e-mail, June 20, 2009.

10. U.S. Department of Veterans Affairs, "Denver Acquisition and Logistics Center Remote Order Entry System (ROES)," http://www.va.gov/EAUTH/ROES/DALC_ROES.asp (accessed October 5, 2009).

11. U.S. Department of Veterans Affairs, "The Denver Acquisition and Logistics Center (DALC) provides Products and Services to Veterans Health Administration Clinics and other Government Agencies Nationally and Disabled Veterans Worldwide," http://www1.va.gov/oamm/_bf/pmo/ALDWebcurrentcatald.pdf (accessed October 5, 2009).

12. U.S. Department of Veterans Affairs, "Guide and Service Dogs," http://www1.va.gov/health/ServiceAndGuideDogs.asp (accessed October 5, 2009).

13. United States of America *ex rel.* Brenda March v. Cochlear Americas, Inc., and Cochlear Limited (District Court for the District of Colorado 2007), Civil Action No. 04-cv-00018-RPM-OES: 11–14.

14. U.S. Department of Justice, Office of Public Affairs, "United States Settles False Claims Act Allegations with Cochlear Americas for $880,000," June 9, 2010, http://www.justice.gov/opa/pr/2010/June/10-civ-673.html (accessed July 28, 2010).

Chapter 4: Sweat, Pump, Recharge, and Glow

1. National Institutes of Health, National Institute of Mental Health, "Anxiety Disorders," http://www.nimh.nih.gov/health/topics/anxiety-disorders/index.shtml (accessed November 16, 2009); National Institute of Mental Health, "Generalized Anxiety Disorder (GAD)," http://www.nimh.nih.gov/health/publications/anxiety-disorders/generalized-anxiety-disorder-gad.shtml (accessed July 20, 2010).

2. Mayo Clinic staff, "Generalized Anxiety Disorder: Lifestyle and Home Remedies," Mayo Foundation for Medical Education and Research, September 11, 2009, http://www.mayoclinic.com/health/generalized-anxiety-disorder/DS00502/DSECTION=lifestyle-and-home-remedies (accessed November 12, 2009).

3. Mayo Clinic staff, "Stress Management: Exercise: Rev Up Your Routine to Reduce Stress," July 23, 2008, http://www.mayoclinic.com/health/exercise-and-stress/SR00036 (accessed November 12, 2009).

4. The President's Council on Physical Fitness and Sports, "Resources: Physical Activity Facts," http://www.fitness.gov/resources_factsheet.htm (accessed November 21, 2009).

5. National Institutes of Health, National Institute on Deafness and Other Communication Disorders, "Can a Dietary Supplement Stave Off Hearing Loss?," February 10, 2009, http://www.nidcd.nih.gov/news/releases/09/02_10_09.htm (accessed November 16, 2009).

6. Cleveland Clinic Miller Family Heart & Vascular Institute, "Heart-Health Benefits of Chocolate Unveiled," http://my.clevelandclinic.org/heart/prevention/nutrition/chocolate.aspx (accessed November 15, 2009).

Chapter 5: To Your Health

1. Karen B. DeSalvo and others, "Predicting Mortality and Healthcare Utilization with a Single Question," *Health Services Research* 40, no. 4 (2005): 1240; Daniel L. McGee and others, "Self-reported Health Status and Mortality in a Multiethnic U.S. Cohort," *American Journal of Epidemiology* 149, no. 1 (1999): 43–44; Joseph T. Ciccolo and others, "Association Between Self-reported Resistance Training and Self-rated Health in a National Sample of U.S. Men and Women," *Journal of Physical Activity & Health* 7, no. 3 (2010): 289.

2. Philip Zazove and others, "The Health Status and Health Care Utilization of Deaf and Hard-of-Hearing Persons," *Archives of Family Medicine* 2, no. 7 (1993): 747–748.

3. Centers for Disease Control and Prevention, National Center for Chronic Disease Prevention and Health Promotion, *Diabetes: Successes and Opportunities for Population-Based Prevention and Control at a Glance*, 2009, http://www.cdc.gov/nccdphp/publications/aag/pdf/diabetes.pdf (accessed March 2, 2009).

4. Agency for Healthcare Research and Quality, Medical Expenditure Panel Survey, custom tabulations of the 2006 Medical Expenditure Panel Survey, Number of People with Care for Selected Conditions by Type of Service, United States (table 1), generated October 12, 2009.

5. Author calculations of 2008 National Health Interview Survey data. See appendix A for technical notes.

6. Author calculations of 2008 National Health Interview Survey data. See appendix A for technical notes.

7. Agency for Healthcare Research and Quality, Medical Expenditure Panel Survey, custom tabulations of the 2007 Medical Expenditure Panel Survey, Mean Expenses per Person with Care for Selected Conditions by Type of Service, United States (table 3a), generated July 19, 2010.

8. J. A. Stevens and others, "The Costs of Fatal and Non-fatal Falls Among Older Adults," *Injury Prevention* 12, no. 5 (2006): 292.

9. American Diabetes Association, "Living with Diabetes: Stress," http://www.diabetes.org/living-with-diabetes/complications/stress.html (accessed July 19, 2010).

10. A.A. Orabi and others, "Cochlear Implant Outcomes and Quality of Life in the Elderly: Manchester Experience Over 13 Years," *Clinical Otolaryngology* 31, no. 2 (2006): 116.

11. Author analysis of 2008 National Health Interview Survey data. See appendix A for technical notes.

Chapter 6: When Silence Isn't Golden

1. Author analysis of 2008 National Health Interview Survey data; see appendix A for technical notes.

2. Author analysis of 2007 National Health Interview Survey data; see appendix A for technical notes.

3. Hearing Industries Association, *A White Paper Addressing the Societal Costs of Hearing Loss and Issues in Third Party Reimbursement*, September 2003, http://www.hearing.org/uploadedFiles/Reimbursement%20White%20Paper%20(12.2008).pdf (accessed July 27, 2010), 2.

4. U.S. Department of Labor, Bureau of Labor Statistics, Inflation Calculator, http://data.bls.gov/cgi-bin/cpicalc.pl (accessed November 15, 2009).

5. Robert I. Field, *Health Care Regulation in America: Complexity, Confrontation, and Compromise* (New York: Oxford University Press, 2007), 76–78.

6. Paul V. McNutt, radio address read into the record on request of Joseph H. Ball on October 23, 1941, 77th Cong., 1st sess., *Congressional Record* 87, pt. 14: A4793.

7. Norton Canfield and Leslie E. Morrissett, "Military Aural Rehabilitation," in *Hearing and Deafness: A Guide for Laymen*, ed. Hallowell Davis, 318–330 (New York: Murray Hill Books, 1947).

8. Ibid., 330–334.

9. U.S. Department of Veterans Affairs, Denver Acquisition and Logistics Center, Veterans Health Information Systems and Technology Architecture data, e-mail message to author, June 20, 2009.

10. Centers for Disease Control and Prevention, National Institute for Occupational Safety and Health, *Work-related Hearing Loss* (NIOSH Publication No. 2001–103: 2001), http://www.cdc.gov/niosh/docs/2001–103/ (accessed November 19, 2009).

11. Beltone, "The Forties," http://www.beltone.com/welcome/history.aspx (accessed September 22, 2009).

12. U.S. Senate, Committee on the Judiciary, Subcommittee on Antitrust and Monopoly, *Prices of Hearing Aids, pursuant to S. Res. 258*, (Senate report no. 2216), October 1, 1962, 87th Cong., 2nd sess., (Washington, DC: GPO, 1962), 113–115.

13. U.S. Senate, Committee on the Judiciary, Subcommittee on Antitrust and Monopoly, *Prices of Hearing Aids: Hearings, pursuant to S. Res. 258*, April 18, 19, 24, 25, and May 16, 1962, 87th Cong., 2nd sess., (Washington, DC: GPO, 1962), 266–270.

14. U.S. Senate, Committee on the Judiciary, April 18, 19, 24, 25, and May 16, 1962, 5.

15. Maurine B. Neuberger, "Don't Listen to Hearing Aid Gyps," September 16, 1965, 89th Cong., 1st sess., *Congressional Record* 111, pt. 28: A5227–5228.

16. U.S. Senate, Committee on the Judiciary, April 18, 19, 24, 25, and May 16, 1962, 11–12.

17. U.S. Senate, "Hearing Aids," October 22, 1965, 89th Cong., 1st sess., Vol. 111, pt. 21, *Congressional Record—Senate*, (Washington, DC: GPO), 28265–28267.

18. Mark Ross, "*Today's Debate: Over-the-Counter (OTC) Hearing Aids,*" http://www.hearingloss.org/magazine/2004SeptOct/RossS004.doc (accessed July 20, 2010): 13. (First published September/October 2004 issue of *Hearing Loss.*)

19. *Transitional Provision on Eligibility of Presently Uninsured Individuals for Hospital Insurance Benefits,* Public Law 89–97, *U.S. Statutes at Large* 79 (1966): 325.

20. U.S. House Subcommittee on Health and Long-Term Care of the Select Committee on Aging, *Medical Appliances and the Elderly: Unmet Needs and Excessive Costs for Eyeglasses, Hearing Aids, Dentures, and Other Devices,* (Washington, DC: GPO, September 1976), xi-xii.

21. U.S. Food and Drug Administration, "Title 21—Food and Drugs, Chapter 1, Subchapter H, Part 801—Hearing Aid Devices: Professional and Patent Labeling and Conditions for Sale," *Federal Register* 42, no. 31 (February 15, 1977): 9286–9296.

22. Ibid., 9288.

23. James Jerger, A Brief Audiological Journey, http://www.audiology.org/Documents/AN2009Handouts/FS111_Jerger.pdf

24. The Academy of Doctors of Audiology, "About the Academy of Doctors of Audiology," http://www.audiologist.org/about-us.pdf (accessed November 19, 2009).

25. American Speech-Language-Hearing Association, "Who are Qualified Providers?," http://asha.org/public/add-benefits/providers.htm (accessed February 15, 2009).

26. Ibid.

27. Council For Clinical Certification in Audiology and Speech-Language Pathology of the American Speech-Language-Hearing Association, *2007 Standards and Implementation Procedures for the Certificate of Clinical Competence in Audiology: Standard I: Degree* (revised March 2009), http://www.asha.org/certification/aud_standards_new.htm (accessed July 19, 2010).

28. Tracy Harding and Susan Paarlberg, "Distance Education Success Fueled by EPAC," *Advance for Audiologists* 9, no. 5 (2007): 79, http://audiology.advanceweb.com/Editorial/Content/PrintFriendly.aspx?CC=169055 (accessed November 19, 2009).

29. American Medical Association, *AMA Scope of Practice Data Series: Audiologists,* (2009): 22–24, http://asha.http.internapcdn.net/asha_vitalstream_com/email/2009/AMAScopeOfPracticeDataSeries.pdf (accessed November 19, 2009).

30. Audiology Foundation of America, *The Au.D. degree: Why it is Needed Now,* April 2004, http://www.audfound.org/files/

AuDdegree.pdf (accessed November 19, 2009); American Speech-Language-Hearing Association, "2009 Public Policy Agenda," http://asha.org/advocacy/briefs-agenda/09PPA.htm (accessed November 19, 2009).

31. Audiology Foundation of America, *Audiology: A Doctoring Profession*, January 2007, http://www.audfound.org/files/AuD Profession.pdf (accessed November 19, 2009).

32. American Academy of Otolaryngology—Head and Neck Surgery, "Numerous Groups Join Ear, Nose, and Throat Doctors in Opposing Dangerous Legislation to Inappropriately Expand Audiologists' Scope of Practice," April 8, 2008, http://www.entnet .org/AboutUs/upload/2008_04_08-HR-1665-letter-news-release.pdf (accessed November 19, 2009).

33. The Hearing Review, "Direct Access to Audiologists Part of ASHA's Lobbying Efforts," April 3, 2007, http://www.hearing review.com/news/2007–04–03_01.asp (accessed September 10, 2009); The Hearing Review, "Direct Access Bill Introduced; AAO-HNS opposes bill, blasts AAA," August 6, 2009, http://www.hearing review.com/issues/articles/2009–08_06.asp (accessed July 19, 2010).

34. American Speech-Language-Hearing Association, "Supply and Demand Resource List for Audiologists," January 2009, http://www.asha.org/uploadedFiles/research/09AudiologySupplyDe mand.pdf (accessed July 19, 2010); 4.

35. Thomas D. Snyder and Sally A. Dillow, U.S. Department of Education National Center for Education Statistics, *Digest of Education Statistics 2009*, Table 275: Bachelor's, master's, and doctor's degrees conferred by degree-granting institutions, by sex of student and discipline division: 2007–08 (Washington, DC: National Center for Education Statistics, 2010), http://nces.ed.gov/programs/di gest/d09/tables/dt09_275.asp (accessed July 19, 2010).

36. Harding and Paarlberg, 79.

37. U.S. Department of Labor, Bureau of Labor Statistics, *Occupational Outlook Handbook, 2010–11 Edition*, December 17, 2009, http://www.bls.gov/oco/ocos085.htm#outlook (accessed July 19, 2010).

38. Kenneth E. Smith, "Think Beyond Hearing Aids to Create Multiple Profit Centers in Your Clinic," *The Hearing Journal* 57, no. 6 (2004): 26.

39. Wayne J. Staab, "Marketing Principles and Application," in *Audiology Practice Management*, 2nd ed., eds. Holly Hosford-Dunn, Ross J. Roeser, and Michael Valente, 112–113, (New York: Thieme Medical Publishers, 2008).

40. Hearing Central LLC, "Hearing Aid Marketing Opportunities: United States Hearing Aid Market," PowerPoint presentation: slides 29–39, summer 2006, updated December 2007 and June 2008, http://www.hearingcentral.com/HearingAidOpportunities.ppt (accessed Aug. 25, 2009).

41. Ibid., slide 40.

42. U.S. Department of Health and Human Services, Food and Drug Administration, "Hearing Aids and Personal Sound Amplifiers: Know the Difference," July 19, 2010, http://www.fda.gov/ForCon sumers/ConsumerUpdates/ucm185459.htm (accessed July 19, 2010).

43. Ibid.

44. Robert Sweetow and David Fabry, "The Great Debate: Is Third-Party Pay Friend or Foe to Audiology?," *The Hearing Journal* 58, no. 9 (2005): 50; Alison M. Grimes and Pauline Casey, "Health Insurance: Should Hearing Aids Be Included?," Audiology Online, May 14, 2001, http://www.audiologyonline.com/articles/pf _article_detail.asp?article_id=287 (accessed November 19, 2009).

45. Gyl A. Kasewurm, "The Case of the Missing Cash," *The Hearing Journal* 59, no. 8 (2006): 46.

46. Judith Nemes, "Third-Party Coverage of Hearing Aids: A Report on Current Initiatives," Sidebar: "Pitfalls of Third-Party Coverage," *The Hearing Journal* 57, no. 7 (2004): 20.

47. Council For Clinical Certification in Audiology and Speech-Language Pathology of the American Speech-Language-Hearing Association, *2007 Standards and Implementation Procedures for the Certificate of Clinical Competence in Audiology: Standard I: Degree* (revised March 2009), http://www.asha.org/certification/aud_standards _new.htm (accessed July 19, 2010).

Chapter 7: Going to the Dogs

1. Claire M. Guest, Glyn M. Collis, and June McNicholas, "Hearing Dogs: A Longitudinal Study of Social and Psychological Effects on Deaf and Hard-of-Hearing Recipients," *Journal of Deaf Studies and Deaf Education* 11, no. 2 (2006): 252–253.

2. International Hearing Dog Inc., "Our Hearing Dog History," http://www.ihdi.org/Program_History.html (accessed July 23, 2010).

3. "A Bill to Provide Financial Assistance to Centers Which Train Dogs to Assist Individuals with Hearing Disabilities; to the Committee on Interstate and Foreign Commerce," HR 12002, 95th Cong., 2d sess., *Congressional Record* 124, pt. 8 (April 11, 1978): H 9695.

4. Assistance Dogs International Inc., "What is ADI Accreditation?," http://www.assistancedogsinternational.org/adiaccreditation.php (accessed November 5, 2009).

5. San Francisco Society for the Prevention of Cruelty to Animals, letter to author dated May 12, 2008.

6. San Francisco Society for the Prevention of Cruelty to Animals, letter to author dated June 11, 2008.

Chapter 8: Learning for a Lifetime

1. Author calculations of 2008 National Health Interview Survey data. See appendix A for technical notes.

2. Jennifer Cheeseman Day and Eric C. Newburger, "The Big Payoff: Educational Attainment and Synthetic Estimates of Work-Life Earnings," *Current Population Reports no. P23–210* (Washington, DC: U.S. Department of Commerce, Bureau of the Census, Economics and Statistics Administration, 2002), 3.

3. Ashley Stephenson, "Student Quits, Cites Disability Services Error," *The Daily Tar Heel*, October 21, 1997.

4. *Laufer v. Board of Governors of the University of North Carolina*, 1:98-CV-00231, U.S. District Court for the Middle District of North Carolina, Durham Division, (1998): 1.

5. Salome Heyward & Associates, *Audit of Critical Elements of a Disability Services Program* (n.d.): 2, 11–14.

Chapter 9: Relationships

1. Aristotle, "Nicomachean Ethics," in *The Complete Works of Aristotle: The Revised Oxford Translation*, vol. 2, ed. Jonathan Barnes, trans. W.D. Ross, revised trans. J.O. Urmson (Princeton, N.J: Princeton University Press, 1984), 1796.

Conclusion

1. Hearing Industries Association, "Meet the Members," http://hearing.org/Content.aspx?id=50 (accessed July 22, 2010).

2. Hearing Industries Association, "The Hearing Aid Tax Credit," *http://hearing.org/Content.aspx?id=44* (accessed July 22, 2010).

3. Author review of Advanced Bionics, "AB Contact Customer Service," http://www.advancedbionics.com/Support_Center/Customer_Support/Contact_Customer_Service.cfm?langid=1 (accessed July 22, 2010); Cochlear Limited, "Cochlear offices," February 5, 2007, http://www.cochlearamericas.com/Support/405.asp (accessed July 22, 2010); and Medical Electronics, "MED-EL Addresses Worldwide,"

http://www.cochlearimplants.com/ENG/US/60_Contact_and
_support/10_Contact_a_MED-EL_office/000_medel_address.asp
(accessed July 22, 2010).

4. Author analysis of companies listed on Hearing Industries Association, "Meet the Members," http://hearing.org/Content
.aspx?id=50 (accessed July 22, 2010).

Appendix A

1. Centers for Disease Control and Prevention, National Center
for Health Statistics, e-mail to the author, December 19, 2008.

Bibliography

The Academy of Doctors of Audiology. "About the Academy of Doctors of Audiology." http://www.audiologist.org/about-us.pdf.

Advanced Bionics. "AB Contact Customer Service." http://www.advancedbionics.com/Support_Center/Customer_Support/Contact_Customer_Service.cfm?langid=1.

Agency for Healthcare Research and Quality, 2006 Medical Expenditure Panel Survey. Custom Tabulations of the Number of People with Care for Selected Conditions by Type of Service, United States (table 1), generated October 12, 2009.

Agency for Healthcare Research and Quality, 2007 Medical Expenditure Panel Survey. Custom Tabulations of Mean Expenses per Person with Care for Selected Conditions by Type of Service, United States (table 3a), generated July 19, 2010.

American Academy of Otolaryngology—Head and Neck Surgery. "Numerous Groups Join Ear, Nose, and Throat Doctors in Opposing Dangerous Legislation to Inappropriately Expand Audiologists' Scope of Practice." News release, April 8, 2008. http://www.entnet.org/AboutUs/upload/2008_04_08-HR-1665-letter-news-release.pdf.

American Diabetes Association. "Living with Diabetes: Stress." http://www.diabetes.org/living-with-diabetes/complications/stress.html.

American Medical Association. "AMA Scope of Practice Data Series: Audiologists." American Medical Association, 2009. http://asha.http.internapcdn.net/asha_vitalstream_com/email/2009/AMAScopeOfPracticeDataSeries.pdf.

American Speech-Language-Hearing Association. "2009 Public Policy Agenda." American Speech-Language-Hearing Association. http://asha.org/advocacy/briefs-agenda/09PPA.htm.

———. "State Insurance Mandates for Hearing Aids." http://www.asha.org/advocacy/state/issues/ha_reimbursement.htm.

———. "Supply and Demand Resource List for Audiologists." January 2009. http://www.asha.org/uploadedFiles/research/09AudiologySupplyDemand.pdf.

———. "Who are Qualified Providers?" http://asha.org/public/add-benefits/providers.htm.

Aristotle. "Nicomachean Ethics." In *The Complete Works of Aristotle: The Revised Oxford Translation.* Vol. 2. Edited by Jonathan Barnes. Translated by W.D. Ross. Revised translation by J. O. Urmson. Princeton, N.J: Princeton University Press, 1984.

ASLInfo.com. "Deaf Time-Line: 1971–1988." http://www.aslinfo.com/trivia4.cfm.

Assistance Dogs International, Inc. "What is ADI Accreditation?" http://www.assistancedogsinternational.org/adiaccreditation.php.

Audiology Foundation of America. *The Au.D. degree: Why it is Needed Now.* Audiology Foundation of America, April 2004. http://www.audfound.org/files/AuDdegree.pdf.

———. *Audiology: A Doctoring Profession.* Audiology Foundation of America, January 2007. http://www.audfound.org/files/AuD Profession.pdf.

Audiology Online. "Federal Employee Hearing Aid Insurance Benefits Take Effect January 1." January 31, 2009. http://www.audiologyonline.com/news/news_detail.asp?news_id=3573.

Bainbridge, Kathleen E., Howard J. Hoffman, and Catherine C. Cowle. "Diabetes and Hearing Impairment in the United States: Audiometric Evidence from the National Health and Nutrition Examination Survey, 1999–2004." *Annals of Internal Medicine* 149 (2008): 1–10.

Battat, Brenda. Letter to the U.S. Department of Education, Office for Civil Rights, December 22, 1997.

Beltone. "The Forties." http://www.beltone.com/welcome/history.aspx.

Bluhm, Gösta Leon, Niklas Berglind, Emma Nordling, and Mats Rosenlund. "Road Traffic Noise and Hypertension." *Occupational and Environmental Medicine* 64 (2007): 122–126.

Boardman, Jed, Bob Grove, Rachel Perkins, and Geoff Shepherd. "Work and Employment for People with Psychiatric Disabilities." *British Journal of Psychiatry* 182 (2003): 467–468.

The British Society of Hearing Aid Audiologists. *Audiological Provision in Europe: A Public-Private Partnership?* February 2005. http://www.hohadvocates.org/europeanreport.pdf.

Bruck, Dorothy, and Ian R. Thomas. "Smoke Alarms for Sleeping Adults Who are Hard-of-Hearing: Comparison of Auditory, Visual, and Tactile Signals." *Ear and Hearing* 30 (2009): 73–80.

Butsch, Richard. *The Making of American Audiences: From Stage to Television, 1750–1990*. Cambridge: Cambridge University Press, 2000.

CBS News.com. "Hearing Loss Now A Military Epidemic," CBS News, March 8, 2008, http://www.cbsnews.com/stories/2008/03/08/health/main3919311.shtml.

Canfield, Norton, and Leslie E. Morrissett. "Military Aural Rehabilitation." In *Hearing and Deafness: A Guide for Laymen*, edited by Hallowell Davis, 318–337. New York: Murray Hill Books, 1947.

Centers for Disease Control and Prevention, National Center for Chronic Disease Prevention and Health Promotion. *Diabetes: Successes and Opportunities for Population-Based Prevention and Control At a Glance, 2009*. National Center for Chronic Disease Prevention and Health Promotion. http://www.cdc.gov/nccdphp/publications/aag/pdf/diabetes.pdf.

Centers for Disease Control and Prevention, National Institute for Occupational Safety and Health. *Work-related Hearing Loss*. NIOSH Publication No. 2001–103, 2001. http://www.cdc.gov/niosh/docs/2001–103.

Chisolm, Theresa Hnath, Carole E. Johnson, Jeffrey L. Danhauer, Laural J. P. Portz, Harvey B. Abrams, Sharon Lesner, Patricia A. McCarthy, and Craig W. Newman. "A Systematic Review of Health-Related Quality of Life and Hearing Aids: Final Report of the American Academy of Audiology Task Force on the Health-Related Quality of Life Benefits of Amplification in Adults." *Journal of the American Academy of Audiology* 18 (2007): 151–183.

Ciccolo, Joesph T., Kelley K. Pettee Gabriel, Caroline Macera, and Barbara E. Ainsworth. "Association Between Self-reported Resistance Training and Self-rated Health in a National Sample of U.S. Men and Women." *Journal of Physical Activity & Health* 7 (2010): 289–298.

Cleveland Clinic Miller Family Heart & Vascular Institute. "Heart-Health Benefits of Chocolate Unveiled." http://my.clevelandclinic.org/heart/prevention/nutrition/chocolate.aspx.

Cochlear Limited. http://www.cochlearamericas.com/Support/405.asp.

Consumer Reports staff. "Hear Well in a Noisy World: Hearing Aids, Hearing Protection & More." *Consumer Reports* 74, no. 7 (2009): 32–37.

Council For Clinical Certification in Audiology and Speech-Language Pathology of the American Speech-Language-Hearing Association. *2007 Standards and Implementation Procedures for the*

Certificate of Clinical Competence in Audiology (rev. March 2009). http://www.asha.org/certification/aud_standards_new.htm.

Crandell, Carl, Terry L. Mills, and Ricardo Gauthier. "Knowledge, Behaviors, and Attitudes About Hearing Loss and Hearing Protection Among Racial/Ethnically Diverse Young Adults." *Journal of the National Medical Association* 96 (2004): 176–186.

Day, Jennifer Cheeseman, and Eric C. Newburger. "The Big Payoff: Educational Attainment and Synthetic Estimates of Work-Life Earnings." *Current Population Reports no. P23–210*. Washington, D.C: Department of Commerce, Bureau of the Census, Economics and Statistics Administration, 2002.

DeSalvo, Karen B., Vincent S. Fan, Mary B. McDonell, and Stephan D. Fihn. "Predicting Mortality and Healthcare Utilization with a Single Question." *Health Services Research* 40 (2005): 1234–1246.

Duke University Center for Demographic Studies, Medical Technology Assessment Working Group. *Assessing the Impact of Medical Technology Innovations on Human Capital: Phase I Final Report (Part G): Effects of Advanced Medical Technologies—Sensory Diseases, Hearing Impairment.* Prepared for the Institute for Medical Technology Innovation, January 31, 2006.

Federal Communications Commission. "Closed Caption Decoder Requirements for Analog Television Receivers." *Code of Federal Regulations*, Title 47, Vol. 1, Sec 15.119, revised October 1, 2005. http://edocket.access.gpo.gov/cfr_2005/octqtr/47cfr15.119.htm.

Federal Communications Commission, Consumer & Governmental Affairs Bureau. "Closed Captioning: FCC Consumer Advisory: Closed Captioning for Digital Television (DTV)." http://www.fcc.gov/cgb/consumerfacts/dtvcaptions.html.

Federal Communications Commission, Consumer & Governmental Affairs Bureau. "Closed Captioning: FCC Consumer Facts." http://www.fcc.gov/cgb/consumerfacts/closedcaption.html.

Field, Robert I. *Health Care Regulation in America: Complexity, Confrontation, and Compromise.* New York: Oxford University Press, 2007.

Grimes, Alison M., and Pauline Casey. "Health Insurance: Should Hearing Aids Be Included?" *Audiology Online*, May 14, 2001. http://www.audiologyonline.com/articles/pf_article_detail.asp?article_id=287.

Guest, Claire M., Glyn M. Collis, and June McNicholas. "Hearing Dogs: A Longitudinal Study of Social and Psychological Effects on Deaf and Hard-of-Hearing Recipients." *Journal of Deaf Studies and Deaf Education* 11 (2006): 252–261.

Harding, Tracy, and Susan Paarlberg. "Distance Education Success Fueled by EPAC." *Advance for Audiologists* 9 (2007): 79. http://audiology.advanceweb.com/Editorial/Content/PrintFriendly.aspx?CC=169055.

Haskell, George B., Douglas Noffsinger, Vernon D. Larson, David W. Williams, Robert A. Dobie, and Janette L. Rogers. "Subjective Measures of Hearing Aid Benefit in the NIDCD/VA Clinical Trial." *Ear and Hearing* 23 (2002): 301–307.

Hearing Central LLC. "Hearing Aid Marketing Opportunities: United States Hearing Aid Market (U.S.A. Hearing Aid Market)." PowerPoint presentation, summer 2006, updated December 2007 and June 2008. http://www.hearingcentral.com/HearingAidOpportunities.ppt.

Hearing Industries Association. "The Hearing Aid Tax Credit," http://hearing.org/Content.aspx?id=44.

———. "Meet the Members," http://hearing.org/Content.aspx?id=50.

———. *A White Paper Addressing the Societal Costs of Hearing Loss and Issues in Third Party Reimbursement.* September 15, 2003. http://www.hearing.org/uploadedFiles/Reimbursement%20White%20Paper%20(12.2008).pdf.

The Hearing Review. "Direct Access to Audiologists Part of ASHA's Lobbying Efforts." *The Hearing Review,* April 3, 2007. http://www.hearingreview.com/news/2007–04–03_01.asp.

———. "Direct Access Bill Introduced; AAO-HNS opposes bill, blasts AAA." *The Hearing Review,* August 6, 2009. http://www.hearingreview.com/issues/articles/2009–08_06.asp.

Heyward, Salome & Associates. *Audit of Critical Elements of a Disability Services Program,* n.d.

Hoffmann, Barbara, Susanne Moebus, Nico Dragano, Stefan Möhlenkamp, Michael Memmesheimer, Raimund Erbel, and Karl-Heinz Jöckel. "Residential Traffic Exposure and Coronary Heart Disease: Results from the Heinz Nixdorf Recall Study." *Biomarkers* 14, no. S1 (2009): 74–78.

Institute of Medicine of the National Academies. *100 Initial Priority Topics for Comparative Effectiveness Research,* 2009. http://www.iom.edu/~/media/Files/Report%20Files/2009/ComparativeEffectivenessResearchPriorities/Stand%20Alone%20List%200f%20100%20CER%20Priorities%20-%20for%20web.pdf.

Integrated Public Use Microdata Series (IPUMS) USA. "The Census of 1850." http://usa.ipums.org/usa/voliii/items1850.shtml.

International Hearing Dog, Inc. "Our Hearing Dog History." http://www.ihdi.org/Program_History.html.

Jerger, James. *A Brief Audiological Journey.* http://www.audiology.org/Documents/AN2009Handouts/FS111_Jerger.pdf.

Kasewurm, Gyl A. "The Case of the Missing Cash." *The Hearing Journal* 59 (2006): 46.

Kirkwood, David H. "Economic Turmoil Threatens to Reverse Recent Growth in the Hearing Aid Market." *The Hearing Journal* 61 (2008): 9–12.

Kisilevsky, B. S., S. M. J. Hains, C. A. Brown, C. T. Lee, B. Cowperthwaite, S. S. Stutzman, M. L. Swansburg, et al. "Fetal Sensitivity to Properties of Maternal Speech and Language." *Infant Behavior & Development* 32 (2009): 59–71.

Lane, Harlan. *When the Mind Hears: A History of the Deaf.* New York: Vintage Books, 1989.

Laufer v. Board of Governors of the University of North Carolina. 1:98-CV-00231. U.S. District Court for the Middle District of North Carolina, Durham Division, 1998.

Mayo Clinic staff. "Generalized Anxiety Disorder: Lifestyle and Home Remedies." Mayo Foundation for Medical Education and Research, September 11, 2009. http://www.mayoclinic.com/health/generalized-anxiety-disorder/DS00502/DSECTION=lifestyle-and-home-remedies.

———. "Stress Management: Exercise: Rev up Your Routine to Reduce Stress." Mayo Clinic, July 23, 2008. http://www.mayoclinic.com/health/exercise-and-stress/SR00036.

McGee, Daniel L., Youlian Liao, Guichan Cao, and Richard S. Cooper. "Self-reported Health Status and Mortality in a Multiethnic US Cohort." *American Journal of Epidemiology* 149, no. 1 (1999): 41–46.

Medical Electronics. *MED-EL Addresses Worldwide.* http://www.cochlearimplants.com/ENG/US/60_Contact_and_support/10_Contact_a_MED-EL_office/000_medel_address.asp.

Medical News Today. "New NHS Focus On Audiology Brings Faster Hearing Aid Treatment." *Medical News Today,* May 21, 2009. http://www.medicalnewstoday.com/articles/150979.php.

National Institutes of Health. "Fact Sheet: Hair Cell Regeneration and Hearing Loss." National Institutes of Health, September 2007. http://www.nih.gov/about/researchresultsforthepublic/Hair.pdf.

National Institutes of Health, National Institute on Deafness and Other Communication Disorders. "Can a Dietary Supplement Stave Off Hearing Loss?" NIDCD media tip sheet, February 10, 2009. http://www.nidcd.nih.gov/news/releases/09/02_10_09.htm.

———. "Cochlear Implants." National Institute on Deafness and Other Communication Disorders, August 31, 2009. http://www.nidcd.nih.gov/health/hearing/coch.htm#c.

———. "Long Description for New Cochlear Implants in 2001." National Institute on Deafness and Other Communication Disorders, April 3, 2008. http://www.nidcd.nih.gov/health/statistics/long-implants.htm.

———. "New Cochlear Implants in 2001." National Institute on Deafness and Other Communication Disorders, June 11, 2008. http://www.nidcd.nih.gov/health/statistics/implants.htm.

———. "Noise: Keeping It Down at Home." National Institute on Deafness and Other Communication Disorders, http://noisyplanet.nidcd.nih.gov/staticresources/materials/Parent Tipsheet_KeepDownatHome.pdf.

National Institutes of Health, National Institute of Mental Health. "Anxiety Disorders," National Institute of Mental Health, November 16, 2009. http://www.nimh.nih.gov/health/topics/anxiety-disorders/index.shtml.

———. "Generalized Anxiety Disorder (GAD)." National Institute of Mental Health, November 16, 2009. http://www.nimh.nih.gov/health/topics/generalized-anxiety-disorder-gad/index.shtml.

Nemes, Judith. "Third-Party Coverage of Hearing Aids: A Report on Current Initiatives (Sidebar: "Pitfalls of Third-Party Coverage"). *The Hearing Journal* 57 (2004): 19–20, 22, 24.

Orabi, A. A., D. Mawman, F. Al-Zoubi, S. R. Saeed, and R. T. Ramsden. "Cochlear Implant Outcomes and Quality of Life in the Elderly: Manchester Experience over 13 Years." *Clinical Otolaryngology* 31 (2006): 116–122.

Prasher, Deepak. "Is There Evidence that Environmental Noise is Immunotoxic?" *Noise & Health* 11 (2009): 151–155.

The President's Council on Physical Fitness and Sports. "Resources: Physical Activity Facts." http://www.fitness.gov/resources_factsheet.htm.

Pugh, Kenneth C. "Health Status Attributes of Older African-American Adults with Hearing Loss." *Journal of the National Medical Association* 96 (2004): 772–779.

Robbins, Gary. "UCI Finds Way to Ease Severe Ringing in the Ears." *Orange County Register*, January 28, 2009.

Ross, Mark. *Today's Debate: Over-the-Counter (OTC) Hearing Aids*. http://www.hearingloss.org/magazine/2004SeptOct/RossS004.doc. (First published September/October 2004 issue of *Hearing Loss*.)

Simpson, John Andrew, and Edmund S. C. Weiner. *The Oxford English Dictionary.* 2nd ed. Vol. 1. Oxford: Clarendon Press, 1989 (reprinted 1991 with corrections, and 1998).

Simpson, John Andrew, and Edmund S. C. Weiner. *The Oxford English Dictionary.* 2nd ed. Vol. 4. Oxford: Clarendon Press, 1989 (reprinted 1991 with corrections, and 1998).

Smith, Kenneth E. "Think Beyond Hearing Aids to Create Multiple Profit Centers in your Clinic." *The Hearing Journal* 57 (2004): 26, 30.

Snyder, Thomas D., and Sally A. Dillow. U.S. Department of Education, National Center for Education Statistics. *Digest of Education Statistics 2009* (NCES 2010–013). Washington, DC: National Center for Education Statistics, 2010. http://nces.ed.gov/programs/digest/d09/tables/dt09_275.asp.

Social Security Administration. "Your Retirement Benefit: How It Is Figured." January 2010. http://www.ssa.gov/pubs/10070.html.

Staab, Wayne J. "Marketing Principles and Application." In *Audiology Practice Management*, 2nd ed. Edited by Holly Hosford-Dunn, Ross J. Roeser, and Michael Valente, 78–127. New York: Thieme Medical Publishers, 2008.

Stephenson, Ashley. "Student Quits, Cites Disability Services Error." *The Daily Tar Heel*, October 21, 1997.

Stevens, J. A., P. S. Corso, E. A. Finkelstein, and T. R. Miller. "The Costs of Fatal and Non-fatal Falls among Older Adults." *Injury Prevention* 12 (2006): 290–295.

Sweetow, Robert, and David Fabry. "The Great Debate: Is Third-party Pay Friend or Foe to Audiology?" *The Hearing Journal* 58 (2005): 46–48, 50.

Time staff. "Television: Larry Hagman: Vita Celebratio Est." *Time*, August 11, 1980, http://www.time.com/time/magazine/article/0,9171,924377,00.html.

Tsakiropoulou, E., I. Konstantinidis, I. Vital, S. Konstantinidou, and A. Kotsani. "Hearing Aids: Quality of Life and Socio-economic Aspects." *Hippokratia* 11 (2007): 183–186.

Tye-Murray, Nancy, Jacqueline L. Spry, and Elizabeth Mauzé. "Professionals with Hearing Loss: Maintaining that Competitive Edge." *Ear and Hearing* 30 (2009): 475–484.

U.S. Census Bureau. "Detailed Data Files: Population Projections for 2000–2050." http://www.census.gov/population/www/projections/usinterimproj/usproj2000–2050.xls.

U.S. Congress. *Congressional Record.* 77th Cong., 1st sess., 1941. Vol. 87, pt. 14. Hon. Paul V. McNutt, radio address read into the record on request of Hon. Joseph H. Ball. Washington, DC: GPO, October 23, 1941.

———. *Congressional Record*. 89th Cong., 1st sess., 1965. Vol. 111, pt. 28. Hon. Maurine B. Neuberger, "Don't Listen to Hearing Aid Gyps." Washington, DC: GPO, September 16, 1965.

———. *Congressional Record*. 95th Cong., 2nd sess., 1978. Vol. 124, pt. 8. "A Bill to Provide Financial Assistance to Centers Which Train Dogs to Assist Individuals with Hearing Disabilities; to the Committee on Interstate and Foreign Commerce." HR 12002. Washington, DC: GPO, April 11, 1978.

———. *The Patient Protection and Affordable Care Act*, Public Law 111–148, 111th Cong., 2d sess. (January 5, 2010).

———. *Transitional Provision on Eligibility of Presently Uninsured Individuals for Hospital Insurance Benefits*. Public Law 89–97, *U.S. Statutes at Large* 79. Washington, DC: GPO, 1966.

U.S. Department of Health and Human Services, Food and Drug Administration. "Guidance for Industry and FDA Staff: Regulatory Requirements for Hearing Aid Devices and Personal Sound Amplification Products." Food and Drug Administration, February 25, 2009. http://www.fda.gov/MedicalDevices/DeviceRegulationandGuidance/GuidanceDocuments/ucm127086.htm.

———. "Hearing Aids and Personal Sound Amplifiers: Know the Difference." July 19, 2010, http://www.fda.gov/ForConsumers/ConsumerUpdates/ucm185459.htm.

———. "Title 21—Food and Drugs, Chapter 1, Subchapter H, Part 801—Hearing Aid Devices: Professional and Patent Labeling and Conditions for Sale." *Federal Register* 42, no. 31, February 15, 1977.

U.S. Department of Justice, Office of Public Affairs. "United States Settles False Claims Act Allegations with Cochlear Americas for $880,000." June 9, 2010. http://www.justice.gov/opa/pr/2010/June/10-civ-673.html.

U.S. Department of Labor, Bureau of Labor Statistics. "Inflation Calculator." http://data.bls.gov/cgi-bin/cpicalc.pl.

———. *Occupational Outlook Handbook, 2010–11 Edition*. Bureau of Labor Statistics, December 17, 2009. http://www.bls.gov/oco/ocos085.htm.

U.S. Department of Transportation, Federal Aviation Administration. "Cochlear Implants Exempt from Rules Regarding Portable Electronic Devices.'" http://www.faa.gov/other_visit/aviation_industry/airline_operators/airline_safety/info/all_infos/media/2007/inF007022.pdf.

U.S. Department of Veterans Affairs. "The Denver Acquisition and Logistics Center (DALC) Provides Products and Services to Veterans Health Administration Clinics and Other Government Agencies Nationally and Disabled Veterans Worldwide." Department of

Veterans Affairs. http://www1.va.gov/oamm/_bf/pmo/ALDWeb currentcatald.pdf.

———. "Denver Acquisition and Logistics Center Remote Order Entry System (ROES)." http://www.va.gov/EAUTH/ROES/DALC_ROES.asp.

———. "Guide and Service Dogs." http://www1.va.gov/health/ServiceAndGuideDogs.asp.

U.S. House Subcommittee on Health and Long-Term Care of the Select Committee on Aging. *Medical Appliances and the Elderly: Unmet Needs and Excessive Costs for Eyeglasses, Hearing Aids, Dentures, and Other Devices.* Washington, DC: GPO, 1976.

U.S. Senate. "Hearing Aids." *Congressional Record—Senate.* 89th Cong., 1st sess. Vol. 111, pt. 21. Washington, DC: GPO, October 22, 1965.

U.S. Senate, Committee on the Judiciary, Subcommittee on Antitrust and Monopoly. *Prices of Hearing Aids: Hearings April 18, 19, 24, 25, and May 16, 1962.* Pursuant to S. Res. 258. 87th Cong., 2nd sess. Washington, DC: GPO, 1962.

———.*Prices of Hearing Aids.* Pursuant to S. Res. 258. (Senate report no. 2216). 87th Cong., 2nd sess. Washington, DC: GPO, October 1,1962.

United States of America ex rel. Brenda March v. Cochlear Americas, Inc, and Cochlear Limited. United States District Court for the District of Colorado, Civil Action No. 04-cv-00018-RPM-OES, 2007.

Walker, Alice. *Possessing the Secret of Joy.* New York: Pocket Books/Simon & Schuster, 1992.

Wallhagen, Margaret I., William J. Strawbridge, Richard D. Cohen, and George A. Kaplan. "An Increasing Prevalence of Hearing Impairment and Associated Risk Factors over Three Decades of the Alameda County Study." *American Journal of Public Health* 87 (1997): 440–442.

World Health Organization. "WHO Calls on Private Sector to Provide Affordable Hearing Aids in Developing World." Press release WHO/34, Jul. 11, 2001. http://who.int/inf-pr-2001/en/pr2001–34.html.

Yordon, Judy E. *Roles in Interpretation.* 2nd ed. Dubuque, IA: Wm C. Brown Publishers, 1989.

Zazove, Philip, Lori C. Niemann, Daniel W. Gorenflo, Craig Carmack, David Mehr, James C. Coyne, and Toni Antonucci. "The Health Status and Health Care Utilization of Deaf and Hard-of-Hearing Persons." *Archives of Family Medicine* 2 (1993): 745–752.

Index

Figures and tables are indicated by f and t following page numbers. Italic page numbers denote illustrations.